THE J

GYNECOLOGY
& OBSTETRICS

THE JOHNS HOPKINS
REVIEW OF
GYNECOLOGY
& OBSTETRICS

Second Edition

Department of Gynecology and Obstetrics
The Johns Hopkins University School of Medicine
Baltimore, Maryland

EDITORS

KIMBERLY B. FORTNER, MD

LINDA M. SZYMANSKI, MD, PhD

EDWARD E. WALLACH, MD

 Wolters Kluwer | Lippincott Williams & Wilkins
Health
Philadelphia · Baltimore · New York · London
Buenos Aires · Hong Kong · Sydney · Tokyo

Acquisitions Editor: Sonya Seigafuse
Managing Editor: Ryan Shaw
Marketing Manager: Kimberly Schonberger
Project Manager: Bridgett Dougherty
Manufacturing Manager: Kathleen Brown
Production Services: Maryland Composition Inc
Printer: RR Donnelley Crawfordsville

Library of Congress Cataloging-in-Publication Data
The Johns Hopkins review of gynecology and obstetrics / editors,
Kimberly B. Fortner, Linda Szymanski, Edward E. Wallach. — 2nd ed.
    p. ; cm.
    Rev. ed. of : Johns Hopkins review of obstetrics & gynecology / Department of
Gynecology and Obstetrics, the Johns Hopkins University School of Medicine,
Baltimore, Md. ; editors, Brandon J. Bankowski, Amy E. Hearne, Edward E. Wallach.
2005.
    Companion to: Johns Hopkins manual of gynecology and obstetrics. 3rd ed. 2007.
    Includes bibliographical references and index.
    ISBN-13: 978-0-7817-6719-4
    ISBN-10: 0-7817-6719-9
    1. Obstetrics—Examinations, questions, etc. 2. Obstetrics—Case studies.
3. Gynecology—Examinations, questions, etc. 4. Gynecology—Case studies.
I. Fortner, Kimberly B. II. Szymanski, Linda. III. Wallach, Edward E., 1933- IV. Johns
Hopkins review of obstetrics & gynecology. V. Johns Hopkins review of gynecology
and oncology. 3rd ed. VI. Title: Review of gynecology and obstetrics.
    [DNLM: 1. Genital Diseases, Female—Problems and Exercises. 2. Gynecology—
Problems and Exercises. 3. Obstetrics—Problems and Exercises. 4. Pregnancy
Complications—Problems and Exercises. WP 18.2 J65 2007]
    RG111.J635 2007
    618.076—dc22

                                                                          2006030154

CONTENTS

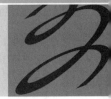

The Preface to the first edition of *The Johns Hopkins Review of Gynecology and Obstetrics* expressed the rationale for its creation. The enthusiasm for just such a text was evident in the rapidity and volume of sales during its first year. It has served as a convenient companion piece for *The Johns Hopkins Manual of Gynecology and Obstetrics* which is currently in its third edition.

To quote from the preface of the first edition, a time-honored method for making the most of any learning experience is to be subjected to a test of knowledge acquired by that experience. Traditionally, this testing which begins in grade school and proceeds through college, graduate school and beyond, has been conducted in the confines of a classroom with the student undergoing quizzes, and final exams. This evaluation process forces that student to review and re-review the material covered by the examination. Even experienced physicians take state licensing board and national board exams as well as continuing certification under this model. Some CME tests cover material from lectures or reading material. However, the ubiquitous examination process is usually not very enjoyable. As physicians, we are fed our knowledge through various sources, but digest and synthesize it though daily clinical experiences. These experiences are truly exercises which make use of the factual and theoretical material which surround us in our day to day practice. As laborious as it is to prepare for and take exams, it is just as highly satisfying to experience the successful clinical application of our knowledge. This book is designed to be a fun-filled, clinically relevant learning experience based on factual material which has been translated to pertain to specific clinical situations and accompanied by a testing process.

The factual material is derived from *The Johns Hopkins Manual of Gynecology and Obstetrics*. This book was originally developed 6 years ago by the house staff and faculty of the Department of Gynecology and Obstetrics of the Johns Hopkins University School of Medicine and Johns Hopkins Hospital. Over 16,000 copies of the first two editions have sold world wide and the 3rd edition is currently available. This companion piece was the brain-child of Dr. Brandon Bankowski who has served as the

Senior House Office editorial Board member of the manual. The current edition of the review book was skillfully supervised by Drs. Kimberly Fortner and Linda Szymanski, now graduates of the residency training program in Gynecology and Obstetrics at Johns Hopkins. Each chapter corresponds to its respective chapter in the manual. The chapters consist of representative cases, as diverse as the practice of Obstetrics and Gynecology itself, which are immediately followed by test questions to challenge the reader and then by a series of feedback statements expressing the rationale for the correct answer.

This Review is tailored to translate the material in the Manual into the language of your clinical mind. As with the Manual, this companion piece is the product of a joint effort by OB/GYN house staff, fellows, and faculty at Johns Hopkins. We hope that you enjoy this learning experience as much as the authors enjoyed preparing if for you, our readers.

Edward E. Wallach, MD
J. Donald Woodruff Professor of Gynecology
Johns Hopkins Medical Institution
Department of Gynecology and Obstetrics

CONTRIBUTORS

Carolyn J. Alexander, MD
Fellow, Division of Reproductive Endocrinology
Department of Gynecology and Obstetrics
Johns Hopkins University School of Medicine
Baltimore, Maryland

Janyne E. Althaus, MD
Division of Maternal Fetal Medicine
Department of Gynecology and Obstetrics
Johns Hopkins University School of Medicine
Baltimore, Maryland

Kristiina Altman, MD
Department of Gynecology and Obstetrics
Johns Hopkins Bayview Medical Center
Baltimore, Maryland

Nancy Arquette, MD
Resident, Department of Gynecology and Obstetrics
Johns Hopkins University School of Medicine
Baltimore, Maryland

Anya Bailis, MD
Resident, Department of Gynecology and Obstetrics
Johns Hopkins University School of Medicine
Baltimore, Maryland

Jacqueline Baselice, MD
Resident, Department of Gynecology and Obstetrics
Johns Hopkins University School of Medicine
Baltimore, Maryland

Karin Blakemore, MD
Director, Maternal-Fetal Medicine
Division of Maternal Fetal Medicine
Johns Hopkins University School of Medicine
Baltimore, Maryland

Anne Burke, MD, MPH
Department of Gynecology and Obstetrics
Johns Hopkins Bayview Medical Center
Baltimore, Maryland

Catherine D. Cansino, MD
Fellow, Contraception, Abortion, and Reproductive Health
Department of Gynecology and Obstetrics
Johns Hopkins Bayview Medical Center
Baltimore, Maryland

David Chang, MD
Resident, Department of Gynecology and Obstetrics
Johns Hopkins University School of Medicine
Baltimore, Maryland

Jennifer E. Cho, MD
Resident, Department of Gynecology and Obstetrics
Johns Hopkins University School of Medicine
Baltimore, Maryland

Natalia Colón, MD
Resident, Department of Gynecology and Obstetrics
Johns Hopkins University School of Medicine
Baltimore, Maryland

Michael Choti, MD, MBA
Jacob C. Handelsman Professor of Surgery
Johns Hopkins Medicine
Baltimore, Maryland

Alice Chung Cootauco, MD
Fellow, Division of Maternal Fetal Medicine
Department of Gynecology and Obstetrics
Johns Hopkins University School of Medicine
Baltimore, Maryland

Geoffrey W. Cundiff, MD
Chair, Department of Obstetrics and Gynecology
University of British Columbia
Vancouver, British Columbia, Canada

Teresa P. Diaz-Montes, MD, MPH
The Kelly Gynecologic Oncology Service
Department of Gynecology and Obstetrics
Johns Hopkins University School of Medicine
Baltimore, Maryland

M. Shoma Datta, MD
Resident, Department of Gynecology and Obstetrics
Johns Hopkins University School of Medicine
Baltimore, Maryland

Sasha Davidson, MD
Resident, Department of Gynecology and Obstetrics
Johns Hopkins University School of Medicine
Baltimore, Maryland

Catherine Eppes, MD
Resident, Department of Gynecology and Obstetrics
Johns Hopkins University School of Medicine
Baltimore, Maryland

Dayna Finkenzeller, MD
Resident, Department of Gynecology and Obstetrics
Johns Hopkins University School of Medicine
Baltimore, Maryland

Kimberly B. Fortner, MD
Faculty, Department of Obstetrics and Gynecology
Associate Clerkship Director
The University of Tennessee Graduate School of Medicine
The University of Tennessee Medical Center
Knoxville, Tennessee

Harold E. Fox, MD
Chairman, Gynecology and Obstetrics
Division of Maternal Fetal Medicine
Department of Gynecology and Obstetrics
Johns Hopkins University School of Medicine
Baltimore, Maryland

Ginger J. Gardner, MD
The Kelly Gynecologic Oncology Service
Department of Gynecology and Obstetrics
Johns Hopkins University School of Medicine
Baltimore, Maryland

Ruchi Garg, MD
Fellow, Gynecologic Oncology
University of Washington School of Medicine
Seattle, Washington

Robert L. Giuntoli, II, MD
The Kelly Gynecologic Oncology Service
Department of Gynecology and Obstetrics
Johns Hopkins University School of Medicine
Baltimore, Maryland

Andrew Goldstein, MD
Division of Gynecologic Specialties
Department of Gynecology and Obstetrics
Johns Hopkins University School of Medicine
Baltimore, Maryland

Katherine Goodrich, MD
Resident, Department of Gynecology and Obstetrics
Johns Hopkins University School of Medicine
Baltimore, Maryland

Ernest M. Graham, MD
Division of Maternal Fetal Medicine
Department of Gynecology and Obstetrics
Johns Hopkins University School of Medicine
Baltimore, Maryland

Isabel Green, MD
Resident, Department of Gynecology and Obstetrics
Johns Hopkins University School of Medicine
Baltimore, Maryland

John Griffith, MD, MPH
Director, Fibroid Center
Division of Gynecologic Specialties
Department of Gynecology and Obstetrics
Johns Hopkins University School of Medicine
Baltimore, Maryland

Matthew Guile, MD
Resident, Department of Gynecology and Obstetrics
Johns Hopkins University School of Medicine
Baltimore, Maryland

Robert E. Gutman, MD
Department of Gynecology and Obstetrics
Center for Pelvic Floor Health
Johns Hopkins Bayview Medical Center
Baltimore, Maryland

Kamal Hamod, MD, MPH
Division of Gynecologic Specialties
Department of Gynecology and Obstetrics
Johns Hopkins University School of Medicine
Baltimore, Maryland

Janice L. Henderson, MD
Division of Maternal Fetal Medicine
Department of Gynecology and Obstetrics
Johns Hopkins University School of Medicine
Baltimore, Maryland

Cynthia J. Holcroft, MD
Division of Maternal Fetal Medicine
Department of Gynecology and Obstetrics
Johns Hopkins University School of Medicine
Baltimore, Maryland

Nancy A. Hueppchen, MD, MSc
Division of Maternal Fetal Medicine
Department of Gynecology and Obstetrics
Johns Hopkins University School of Medicine
Baltimore, Maryland

K. Joseph Hurt, MD
Resident, Department of Gynecology and Obstetrics
Johns Hopkins University School of Medicine
Baltimore, Maryland

Amy Johnson, MD
Department of Obstetrics and Gynecology
University of Connecticut School of Medicine
Hartford, Connecticut

Valerie Jones, MD
Resident, Department of Gynecology and Obstetrics
Johns Hopkins University School of Medicine
Baltimore, Maryland

Jeremy King, MD
Fellow, Division of Reproductive Endocrinology
Department of Gynecology and Obstetrics
Johns Hopkins University School of Medicine
Baltimore, Maryland

Jennifer Kulp, MD
Resident, Department of Gynecology and Obstetrics
Johns Hopkins University School of Medicine
Baltimore, Maryland

Joel Larma, MD
Resident, Department of Gynecology and Obstetrics
Johns Hopkins University School of Medicine
Baltimore, Maryland

Christopher W. Lipari, MD
Fellow, Division of Reproductive Endocrinology
Department of Gynecology and Obstetrics
Johns Hopkins University School of Medicine
Baltimore, Maryland

Pamela Lipsett, MD
Professor, Surgery, ACCM and Nursing
Surgical Critical Care Fellowship Director
Department of Surgery and Surgical Sciences
Johns Hopkins Medicine
Baltimore, Maryland

Colleen McCormick, MD
Fellow, The Kelly Gynecologic Oncology Service
Department of Gynecology and Obstetrics
Johns Hopkins University School of Medicine
Baltimore, Maryland

Thao Nguyen, MD
Fellow, Urogynecology and Reconstructive Pelvic Surgery
Department of Obstetrics and Gynecology
University of North Carolina-Chapel Hill
Chapel Hill, North Carolina

Mary Ellen Pavone, MD
Resident, Department of Gynecology and Obstetrics
Johns Hopkins University School of Medicine
Baltimore, Maryland

Donald H. Penning, MD, MSc, FRCP
Department of Anesthesiology and Critical Care Medicine
Department of Gynecology and Obstetrics
Director, Division of Obstetric, Regional & Acute Pain Anesthesia
Johns Hopkins University School of Medicine
Baltimore, Maryland

Scott M. Petersen, MD
Fellow, Division of Maternal Fetal Medicine
Department of Gynecology and Obstetrics
Johns Hopkins University School of Medicine
Baltimore, Maryland

Julie Phillips, MD
Resident, Department of Gynecology and Obstetrics
Johns Hopkins University School of Medicine
Baltimore, Maryland

Scott C. Purinton, MD, PhD
Resident, Department of Gynecology and Obstetrics
Johns Hopkins University School of Medicine
Baltimore, Maryland

Francisco Rojas, MD
Johns Hopkins Community Physicians
Department of Gynecology and Obstetrics
Johns Hopkins University School of Medicine
Baltimore, Maryland

Brenda Ross, MD
Division of Maternal Fetal Medicine
Department of Gynecology and Obstetrics
Johns Hopkins University School of Medicine
Baltimore, Maryland

Kristy Ruis, MD
Resident, Department of Gynecology and Obstetrics
Johns Hopkins University School of Medicine
Baltimore, Maryland

Eli A. Rybak, MD, MPH
Department of Obstetrics and Gynecology and Women's Health
Albert Einstein College of Medicine
Montefiore Medical Center
Bronx, New York

Alexander Simopoulos, MD
Laser Vaginal Rejuvenation Institute of Los Angeles
Los Angeles, California

Marium H. Smith, MD
Resident, Department of Gynecology and Obstetrics
Johns Hopkins University School of Medicine
Baltimore, Maryland

Linda M. Szymanski, MD, PhD
Department of Obstetrics and Gynecology
University of South Carolina School of Medicine
Columbia, South Carolina

Edward Tanner, MD
Resident, Department of Gynecology and Obstetrics
Johns Hopkins University School of Medicine
Baltimore, Maryland

Edward Trimble, MD, MPH
The Kelly Gynecologic Oncology Service
Department of Gynecology and Obstetrics
Johns Hopkins University School of Medicine
Baltimore, Maryland
Head, Gynecologic Cancer Therapeutics
National Cancer Institute
Bethesda, Maryland

Nikos Vlahos, MD
Division of Reproductive Endocrinology
Department of Gynecology and Obstetrics
Johns Hopkins University School of Medicine
Baltimore, Maryland

Frank R. Witter, MD
Medical Director of Labor and Delivery
Division of Maternal Fetal Medicine
Department of Gynecology and Obstetrics
Johns Hopkins University School of Medicine
Baltimore, Maryland

Melissa Yates, MD
Resident, Department of Gynecology and Obstetrics
Johns Hopkins University School of Medicine
Baltimore, Maryland

Howard Zacur, MD, PhD
Theodore and Ingrid Professor of Reproductive Endocrinology
Director, REI Fellowship Program
Division of Reproductive Endocrinology
Department of Gynecology and Obstetrics
Johns Hopkins University School of Medicine
Baltimore, Maryland

1

Primary Care

Kimberly B. Fortner and Harold E. Fox

1. In regards to leading causes of death by age group for both men and women, all of the following statements are true *except:*

A. Congenital anomalies are the leading cause of death in children ages 1 to 4.

B. Unintentional injury, homicide, and suicide are the top three causes of death for ages 15 to 34.

C. Cancer is the leading cause of death for ages 45 to 64.

D. Despite the availability of vaccinations, influenza and pneumonia are still in the top five causes of death for age 65 and older.

A Congenital anomalies are the leading cause of death in infants less than age 1. By age 1, unintentional injury becomes the leading cause of death and remains the leading cause until age 45! Cancer is the number two cause of death for ages 5 to 14 and ages 35 to 45, but it becomes the leading cause of death for ages 45 to 64. For individuals age 65 and older, the causes of death are heart disease, cancer, stroke, chronic respiratory disease, influenza, and pneumonia. The CDC recommends vaccination against pneumococcal pneumonia at age 65 and annual vaccination against influenza starting at age 50.

2. Obesity is a major health problem in the United States. Please select the *best* statement with respect to this health issue.

A. Obesity is defined as having a body mass index (BMI) of 35 or greater.

B. One fifth of U.S. women are obese.

C. Obesity increases the risk of developing hypertension, diabetes, infertility, heart disease, gallbladder disease, and several forms of cancer.

D. The physician's role is not to encourage weight loss due to embarrassment for the patient.

C Obesity is defined as BMI of greater than 30. Unfortunately, over one-third of U.S. women are obese, with the highest prevalence reaching 49% in African American women. Obesity imposes numerous comorbidities not limited to the risk of developing hypertension, diabetes, infertility, heart disease, gallbladder disease, and uterine and colon cancer. Other risks include gout, osteoarthritis, elevated cholesterol, insulin resistance, reflux disease, and sleep apnea. Unfortunately, the health care provider stays silent too often with obese patients and does not help address the problem of weight. The surgeon general's call to action encourages everyone to view obesity not as a problem of appearance, but a problem of health (1).

3. Which of the following patients is at *greatest* risk for developing coronary artery disease?

A. A 60-year-old woman who is not on hormone replacement therapy with an LDL of 130 mg/dL

B. A 60-year-old woman who is not on hormone replacement therapy with hypertension and an LDL of 100 mg/dL

C. A 50-year-old, nonsmoking, healthy woman with a family history of a myocardial infarction in her mother at age 55 and an LDL of 100 mg/dL

D. A 60-year-old woman who smokes and has an LDL of 140 mg/dL and an HDL of 25 mg/dL

D The woman described in choice D has three risk factors for the development of coronary artery disease—her age, smoking, and very low high-density lipoprotein (HDL), in addition to her elevated low-density lipoprotein (LDL) cholesterol, making her the most concerning patient on the list. The scenario described in choice A relates one risk factor (increased age) but with a well-controlled LDL. For primary prevention of coronary heart disease, the treatment goal is to achieve an LDL cholesterol level of less than 160 mg/dL in patients with only one risk factor. Choice B has two risk factors, but her LDL is certainly less than the recommended 130 mg/dL. The patient described in choice C has a family history component but a very well-controlled LDL.

4. Which of the following women is *least* likely to necessitate testing for diabetes?

A. A 50-year-old with a BMI of 30

B. A 45-year-old Hispanic American with a history of gestational diabetes

C. A 40-year-old with hypertension, elevated triglycerides, and history of delivering a 10-pound infant.

D. A 35-year-old who has a second cousin with diabetes diagnosed at age 40.

D A 35-year-old woman with a remote family history would be lower on the list to test for diabetes than the other scenarios presented. Diabetes testing should be considered in all individuals at age 45 and older; if results are normal, screening should be initiated every three years unless the patient has other risk factors. Testing should be done at earlier ages or more frequently if the patient:

- Has a BMI>27
- Has first-degree family relative with diabetes
- Is a member of a high-risk ethnic population
- Delivered a baby weighing more than 9 pounds or has been diagnosed with gestational diabetes mellitus
- Has been diagnosed with hypertension
- Has an HDL cholesterol level of 35 mg/dL or lower or a triglyceride level of 250 mg/dL or higher or both
- Previously had impaired glucose tolerance or impaired fasting glucose

References

1. Office of the Surgeon General. The Surgeon General's call to action to prevent and decrease overweight and obesity. Rockville, MD: U.S. Department of Health and Human Services, Public Health Service, Office of the Surgeon General, 2001.

2

Breast Disease

Isabel Green and Michael Choti

1. All of the following are true regarding breast anatomy, *except:*

A. Cooper's suspensory ligaments are fibrous bands of support that connect the deep pectoral fascia to the superficial pectoral fascia.

B. The principal blood supply to the breast is the lateral thoracic artery, and the associated lymphatics mirror the principal blood supply and drain primarily to the axilla (97%).

C. The internal mammary nodes receive bilateral lymphatic drainage from the breasts, and therefore are potential sites of metastasis.

D. The breast tissue is broken up into quadrants, and the most common location for breast cancer is the upper outer quadrant.

B The principal blood supply to the breast is the *internal mammary artery.* This artery comprises two-thirds of the blood supply. The *lateral thoracic artery* supplies only the upper outer quadrant of the breast (one-third). Unlike the majority of organs in the body, the lymphatics and the blood supply to the breast are not parallel. The majority of drainage (97%) is to the axillary nodes, with the remainder draining to the internal mammary nodes. The internal mammary nodes do receive bilateral drainage from the breasts and are a potential site for metastasis from the contralateral breast.

2. A 47-year-old multiparous patient presents to your office and reports finding a hard lump in her left breast on self breast examination for the past 2 weeks. She denies any associated breast pain and believes the lump was not present in the past. She is concerned because her neighbor was recently diagnosed with breast cancer. On examination you note bilateral, symmetric breasts, no palpable masses, no skin changes, normal-appearing nipples, and no lymphadenopathy. Her last mammography was 16 months ago and normal. Your next step in her management is:

A. Diagnostic mammography

B. Ultrasound

C. Screening mammography

D. Re-examination in 1 month

E. Reassurance and return for annual examination

A Clinical breast exam has a sensitivity of approximately 54%. A breast mass reported by the patient should undergo evaluation even it fails to be appreciated on examination. Diagnostic (not screening) mammography is recommended in any woman over age 35 with a breast mass. Ultrasound is useful in women under age 35, those with breast implants, or those on hormone replacement therapy (HRT). Cancerous lesions are typically single, hard, immobile, greater than 2 cm, and have irregular margins. The majority are painless, although 10% may show some symptoms of discomfort. Failure to diagnose breast cancer remains at the top of the list for claims of malpractice, and reassurance is not sufficient evaluation for this patient. According to the Physician Insurers Association of America's Breast Cancer Study, the most common reasons for lawsuits against obstetrician-gynecologists were "physical findings failed to impress" and "failure to refer to specialist for biopsy." Physicians must be prepared to fully evaluate, address, and educate patients regarding their concerns.

3. A 28-year-old woman presents as a new patient for an annual exam. During your history taking she reports a positive family history for breast cancer. On further questioning, she reports breast cancer in her mother, diagnosed at age 52, as well as her maternal aunt at age 58. She denies any other history of breast cancer, ovarian cancer, or colon cancer. Given her history, current recommendations include testing for BRCA1 and BRCA2, in addition to routine mammography screening starting at age 40, self breast exam, and clinical breast exams.

A. True

B. False

> **B** Family history is a very important portion of the annual exam. Family history does confer an increased risk of breast cancer when referring to a **premenopausal** breast cancer history in **first-degree** relatives. This patient's family history is of postmenopausal breast cancer in a first-degree relative and postmenopausal breast cancer in a second-degree relative. The routine screening recommendation would apply, and mammography every 1 to 2 years from ages 40 to 49, followed by annual mammography after age 50. Although clinical breast exams have a sensitivity of 54%, approximately 5% of breast cancers are missed by mammography and detected by clinical breast examination alone. Clinical breast exams are currently recommended annually by ACOG. Guidelines for self breast examination are controversial; however, routine teaching by health providers is recommended. BRCA1 and BRCA2 are tumor suppressor genes with autosomal dominant inheritance. They account for only 5% of all breast cancer diagnoses but do confer a greater than 50% lifetime risk. Patients with a family history of **premenopausal** breast cancer should be referred for genetic counseling and testing.

4. A 25-year-old woman delivered a healthy infant by vaginal delivery 2 weeks previously without complication. She has been breast-feeding since delivery. She presents to your office complaining of severe right-sided breast pain. She also reports symptoms of chills and muscle aches for 2 days. On examination you note an erythematous, indurated area on the right breast, tender and warm to the touch. You recommend all of the following, *except:*

A. Prescription of dicloxacillin (500 mg by mouth four times a day for 10 days)

B. Incision and drainage with culturing if the symptoms worsen

C. Avoidance of breast-feeding from the affected breast until resolution of the infection

D. Treatment with ibuprofen for pain

C Mastitis is an acute cellulitis of the breast, which occurs more commonly in the lactating woman and is termed *puerperal mastitis*. The differential diagnosis includes duct occlusion (without infection), breast abscess, and, rarely, breast cancer. The infection occurs around the duct system and presents with a wedge-shaped pattern over a portion of skin. If not treated promptly it can lead to an abscess, which is fluctuant and less well demarcated. An abscess would require incision and drainage, with culturing to guide antibiotic treatment.

The most common causal organism is *Staphylococcus aureus*, as well as *Streptococcus* and *Escherichia coli*. Treatment usually consists of a trial of a beta-lactam antibiotic (dicloxacillin or cloxacillin) for at least 10 days to prevent relapse. If the infection does not improve over 24 to 48 hours, the antibiotic can be broadened (usually cephalexin or Augmentin). Recurrent mastitis or mastitis that does not respond to appropriate antibiotics should raise the suspicion for breast cancer and prompt biopsy.

Perhaps more important than antibiotic treatment is continued emptying of the affected breast. If this cannot be achieved through breast-feeding alone, pumping or manual expression should be encouraged. Warm compresses, in addition to ibuprofen, can also be recommended for improvement of symptoms.

In contrast, *nonpuerperal mastitis* is usually a polymicrobial infection, and treatment should include clindamycin or metronidazole, in addition to the beta-lactam antibiotic. These women are typically not ill appearing. The threshold for biopsy is much lower, particularly in the elderly patient. In addition, the patient should be up-to-date on mammography as part of her treatment plan.

5. A 36-year-old nulliparous patient presents for her annual exam. On questioning she reports intermittent spontaneous nipple discharge, which she has noticed on her brassiere for the past month. She takes only a daily multivitamin. She denies any recent trauma to either breast and does not have excess breast stimulation or irritating brassieres.

Please match the findings on examination to your recommended workup; an answer may be used more than once.

A. Right-sided discharge, appears clear but noted to be guaiac-positive on smear. No palpable mass or lymphadenopathy. Remainder of history and exam are normal.

B. Bilateral milky discharge and visual field deficit are noted on examination. Patient reports new onset headaches. No palpable mass or lymphadenopathy, and remainder of history and exam is normal.

C. Bilateral milky discharge, normal visual fields. No palpable mass or lymphadenopathy. Hyporeflexic on examination of patellar reflexes. Patient reports 15-pound weight gain in past year.

D. Left-sided discharge, clear and guaiac negative. Small mass palpated in upper outer quadrant, firm approximately 1 to 2 cm in size, not painful on examination. Remainder of history and physical examination are normal.

E. Bilateral milky discharge, normal visual fields. Remainder of examination and history are normal.

1. Send prolactin, TSH, mammography.

2. Order mammography and refer to surgery consult.

3. Send fluid for cytology and refer to surgery consult.

4. Send prolactin, TSH, mammography, CT scan/MRI.

5. Encourage avoidance of nipple stimulation and return in 1 month.

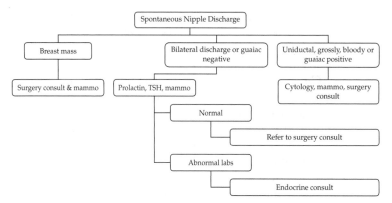

Figure 2.1. Algorithm for evaluation of nipple discharge.

A-3; B-4; C-1; D-2; E-1

The patient describes symptoms of nipple discharge (Fig. 2.1).

Nipple discharge can be divided into categories based on the following factors: **laterality, spontaneous** or **expressed, bloody** (**gross** or **on guaiac**), and if noted to have **associated symptoms** or **mass.** In general, nipple discharge can be either physiologic, pathologic, or due to galactorrhea.

Physiologic discharge is usually **unilateral** and **nonspontaneous.** If she had presented with these symptoms, and had a normal physical examination, no further workup would have been needed. None of the previously mentioned cases fit this description, and, as such, re-examination in 1 month would have been an inadequate evaluation for any of the circumstances (option 5).

Patient A has **unilateral bloody discharge.** Guaiac testing is important to detect subtle bloody fluid that may appear grossly normal. Bloody fluid requires further evaluation with **cytology,** which will assist in identifying proliferative lesions from inflammatory ones (negative cytology). This type of **pathologic discharge** can be caused by **carcinoma, intraductal papilloma (usually straw colored), duct ectasia, and fibrocystic changes.** In addition to cytology, **bilateral mammography** should be performed and **referral to a breast surgeon** for interpretation of cytology and further workup. The finding of a palpable mass, even with negative cytology and in the absence of associated symptoms or findings, should prompt mammography and referral to a breast surgeon for possible biopsy (**patient D**).

Galactorrhea is milk production unrelated to nursing or pregnancy and is typically a bilateral, multiduct discharge with a milky character. Several endocrine abnormalities give rise to galactorrhea and can be associated with amenorrhea (dopamine inhibitors, hypothalamic/pituitary disease, hypothyroid, chronic renal failure). **Patient C** is not taking any additional medications (dopamine inhibitors, oral contraceptives) that may cause galactorrhea, and she does not report a recent history of trauma or stimulation.

The routine endocrine workup for galactorrhea includes sending a TSH and a prolactin level. These should be ordered even in the absence of associated symptoms or findings (**patient E**).

Pituitary adenomas may be associated with new onset headaches, visual field deficits, and an elevated prolactin level. In the absence of symptoms, a CT scan or MRI is not indicated unless the prolactin level returns as elevated. Prolactin levels may be falsely elevated after meals or with diurnal variation, and a repeat test may be required. **Patient B** is noted to have visual field deficits, and a CT scan or MRI should be ordered as part of the initial evaluation.

3

Critical Care

Catherine D. Cansino and Pamela Lipsett

1. A 54-year-old woman is diagnosed with stage IIB endometrial cancer after staging laparotomy. Her past medical history is significant for hypertension controlled with nifedipine. Preoperative EKG, CXR, and stress test showed no abnormalities. Postoperative blood pressure readings ranged from 106 to 118/60 to 72 mm Hg, and pulse readings ranged from 88 to 96 bpm. During her hospital course, she received analgesics and antiemetics as needed and was advanced to a regular diet without complications. On postoperative day 3, she was discharged home in a stable condition. Six days after discharge, she was found unconscious in her home by a family member and was immediately brought to the hospital. She was pronounced dead upon arrival, and autopsy showed evidence of a massive myocardial infarction. Which of the following interventions would have been beneficial in this patient to prevent the subsequent outcome?

A. Preoperative cardiac catheterization
B. Perioperative telemetry
C. Perioperative diuretic administration
D. Perioperative beta-blocker administration

D Several studies have shown that perioperative beta-blockade for heart rate control decreases morbidity and mortality in patients with known cardiac risk factors who undergo noncardiac surgery. Preoperative cardiac catheterization and perioperative telemetry are unnecessary in patients with controlled hypertension and have no evidence of ischemia or arrhythmia on preoperative noninvasive diagnostic studies. Although calcium channel blockade for blood pressure control may need to be restarted outside of the immediate perioperative period, no studies show that administration of previous antihypertensive agents, other than beta-blockers, is beneficial.

2. A 60-year-old woman undergoes an abdominal hysterectomy for benign indications and is discharged after an uncomplicated hospital course on postoperative day 2. She presents to the hospital 9 days after hospital discharge and is noted to have a pelvic abscess above the vaginal cuff diagnosed by computed tomography (CT) in the emergency department. Her past medical history is significant for uncontrolled hypertension, uncontrolled diabetes, and chronic renal insufficiency. On admission, laboratory values are as follows: WBC 13,900/mm^3, hemoglobin 10.4 g/dL, hematocrit 32.6%, neutrophils 87%, creatinine 1.8 mg/dL. She is started on piperacillin/tazobactam 2.25 g intravenously (IV) every 6 hours (renal dose). On hospital day 2, the patient has begun to defervesce but is noted to have the following renal function: creatinine 2.6 mg/dL. What is the most likely etiology?

   A. Inappropriate antibiotic dose
   B. Use of radiographic contrast agent
   C. Acetaminophen toxicity
   D. Pre-existing medical conditions

   B Patients with known renal insufficiency who then receive a radiographic contrast agent may suffer from further reduction in renal function. Other susceptible populations are those who receive high doses of contrast agents and patients who concomitantly receive other nephrotoxic medications. Contrast-induced nephropathy may be caused by the production of reactive oxygen species. Prophylactic administration of the antioxidant acetylcysteine, along with intravenous hydration, has been shown to prevent the reduction in renal function induced by agents used in CT. A recent study also suggests that hydration with sodium bicarbonate, in comparison to normal saline before administration of contrast, may be beneficial as well. In many hospitalized patients the need for IV contrast is urgent and thus bicarbonate therapy may be preferred in at-risk patients.

   The antibiotic regimen given was an appropriate dose given the patient's baseline renal function. Although a nonnephrotoxic antibiotic may have been more appropriate for this patient, no clear evidence shows that piperacillin/tazobactam alone acutely caused a further decline in the patient's renal function. Considering the patient's hospitalization status and controlled medication administration, acetaminophen toxicity is unlikely. Furthermore, symptoms of acetaminophen intoxication, for example, lethargy, pallor, and vomiting, would be evident before laboratory of evidence of nephrotoxicity. The further decline in renal function from the patient's baseline cannot be explained by her pre-existing medical problems and warrants further investigation.

3. A 54-year-old woman with stage IIIC ovarian cancer complains of nausea and fatigue. Her last chemotherapy treatment was 1 month ago. Laboratory data show sodium 122 mEq/L, plasma osmolality 200 mosm/L, urine osmolality 350 mosm/kg, urine sodium 45mEq/L. Syndrome of inappropriate ADH secretion (SIADH) is suspected. She is aggressively resuscitated with normal saline. The next day she is noted to be lethargic, disoriented, and hyperreflexic. Laboratory data reveals resolution of hyponatremia with serum sodium level of 138 mEq/L. What is the most likely etiology of the patient's condition?

   A. Overcorrection of hyponatremia

   B. Insufficient hydration for treatment of SIADH

   C. Side effects of chemotherapy

   D. Brain metastases

   A SIADH is primarily treated by water restriction. Secondary to rapid correction of SIADH-induced hyponatremia with isotonic solution, the patient developed central pontine myelinolysis. Symptoms can be reversed, in some cases, by discontinuing saline infusion and administering hypotonic fluids. In this vignette, toxicity from chemotherapeutic agents is unlikely because the patient is remote from her last treatment and laboratory data support an underlying condition. Insufficient data prevents support of brain metastases.

4. A healthy 26-year-old woman delivered a full-term, viable neonate 8 days ago by cesarean delivery secondary to nonre-

assuring fetal status. Her postoperative course was complicated by endomyometritis that resolved upon administration
of intravenous antibiotics. She returns to Labor and Delivery
with fever and diarrhea. She is subsequently admitted to the
hospital and intravenously hydrated with lactated Ringer's solution. A fecal sample is sent to the laboratory to determine
the presence of *Clostridium difficile* toxin. Meanwhile, laboratory data reveal sodium 136 mEq/L, potassium 3.2 mEq/L,
chloride 94 mEq/L, BUN 10 mg/dL, creatinine 0.8 mg/dL.
The patient is given a potassium chloride infusion of 60 mEq.
On hospital day 2, laboratory findings include sodium 138
mEq/dL, potassium 3.3 mEq/L, chloride 101 mEq/L. Why
does the patient continue to be hypokalemic, despite potassium replacement?

A. Inadequate potassium replacement

B. Inadequate sodium replacement

C. Inadequate magnesium replacement

D. Persistent diarrhea

> **C** Despite persistent diarrhea, this patient is adequately
> hydrated with potassium-containing isotonic solution and
> an appropriate dose of potassium replacement; hy-
> pokalemia should be expected to resolve. However, hypo-
> magnesemia promotes urinary potassium excretion, there-
> fore magnesium replacement should be administered in all
> patients with hypokalemia and normal renal function. In
> treating hypokalemia, one can expect an approximate 0.1-
> mEq/dL rise in the serum potassium level for every 10
> mEq of potassium administered. The plasma potassium
> level is not affected by the plasma sodium levels in patients
> with normal renal function.

5. A 68-year-old woman with recurrent stage IIIB cervical cancer
is brought to the emergency room by family members secondary
to somnolence. A recent outpatient CT scan shows large central
disease refractory to radiation therapy. Laboratory values reveal WBC 10,900/mm^3, hemoglobin 9.1 mg/dL, hematocrit
28.4%, platelets 165,000/mm^3, sodium 145 mEq/L, potassium
6.0 mEq/L, chloride 95 mEq/L, carbon dioxide 32 mEq/L, BUN
35 mg/dL, creatinine 3.2 mg/dL, arterial pH 7.29, PCO$_2$ 30 mm
Hg, PO$_2$ 80 mm Hg, bicarbonate 28 mEq/L. What is the most
likely etiology of the patient's condition?

A. Anemia of chronic disease
B. Urinary tract infection
C. Uremia
D. Overmedication with narcotics

C This patient suffers from uremia caused by distal obstruction secondary to extensive pelvic disease and consequent metabolic acidosis with an increased anion gap [anion gap = $(Na^+ + K^+) - (Cl^- + HCO_3^-)$]. Consider other causes of increased anion gap acidosis (mnemonic MUDPILES): methanol, uremia, diabetic ketoacidosis, paraldehyde, isoniazid, infection, lactic acidosis, ethylene glycol, salicylates. Although the other options may cause somnolence, the severity of the disease relevant to the laboratory findings does not correlate with these conditions.

4

Preconception Counseling and Prenatal Care

Francisco Rojas and Karin Blakemore

1. A 25-year-old gravida 1 para 0, with an unremarkable past medical history but irregular menstrual cycles, presents at your office to start prenatal care. An ultrasound confirms viable intrauterine gestation and crown-rump length (CRL) compatible with 6 weeks. Maternal hematocrit is 33%, and other initial laboratory results are within normal limits. She is concerned because she did not take vitamin and mineral supplementation before this pregnancy. You advise her to start taking:

   A. Prenatal vitamins
   B. Prenatal vitamins and 1.0 mg folate daily
   C. Prenatal vitamins and 4.0 mg folate daily
   D. Prenatal vitamins and 1,200 mg of calcium daily
   E. Prenatal vitamins, 4.0 mg folate, and 1,200 mg of calcium daily

   D Dietary allowances for most minerals and vitamins increase with pregnancy. All of these nutrients, with the exception of iron, are supplied adequately by a well-balanced diet. However, prenatal vitamins contain only 250 mg of calcium, and patients who do not receive adequate dairy products sometimes cannot meet the prenatal daily requirement of 1,200 mg of calcium. Many prenatal vitamins have 1 mg of folic acid, enough to cover the requirements for patients without history of a previous infant with neural tube defects (NTDs) or patients not taking carbamazepine or valproic acid. On the other hand, mothers with a positive history of a pregnancy with an open NTD, or women taking carbamazepine or valproic acid will need to take 4 mg per day of folic acid at least 4 weeks before conception and during the first trimester.

2. A 26-year-old nulliparous patient comes to your office with her husband and establishes that her last menstrual period was 6 weeks ago. She received measles, mumps, rubella (MMR) vaccine and hepatitis-B-recombinant vaccine 3 weeks ago. The patient has been taking vitamins and folic acid. Both parents are healthy with noncontributory past medical histories. After a complete evaluation you confirm an intrauterine viable pregnancy. You advise this couple all of the following, *except:*

   A. She can complete the hepatitis-B-vaccine protocol during the first and second trimester without risk.

   B. Congenital rubella infection is associated with deafness, persistent ductus arteriosus, mental retardation, cataracts, and IUGR, among other abnormalities.

   C. She should consider termination of this pregnancy because of the high risk of congenital rubella.

   D. Measles may increase the risk of spontaneous abortion, preterm birth, and maternal morbidity.

   E. Measles, mumps, rubella vaccine can be given to children of pregnant women.

   C Despite theoretic risks, no case of congenital rubella syndrome has ever been reported after rubella immunization within 3 months before conception or early in pregnancy. Even though the risk of complications is low, the current recommendation is to avoid pregnancy for at least 28 days after receiving a rubella-containing vaccine. The same rule applies to other live-attenuated-virus vaccines. Recombinant hepatitis B is a noninfectious vaccine and is safe during pregnancy. Measles, mumps, and rubella vaccine can be given to children of pregnant women because no evidence shows that someone who has recently been vaccinated can transmit the viruses.

3. A 24-year-old gravida 2 para 1001 at 14 weeks of gestation, a smoker, is brought by the police to the emergency room. Her toxicology screen was positive for cocaine, marijuana, and alcohol. A previous toxicology evaluation several weeks ago on the same patient was positive for cocaine and heroin. She expresses the desire to quit using drugs. After a complete social assessment and an appointment at the rehabilitation center, you explain to the patient all of the following, *except:*

A. Cocaine might produce urinary and cardiac malformations, IUGR, and abruptio placentae.

B. Treatment with methadone is associated with improved pregnancy outcomes.

C. Tetrahydrocannabinol is a potent teratogen.

D. Fetal alcohol syndrome is characterized by fetal and post-natal growth retardation, facial dysmorphology, and CNS dysfunction.

E. Smoking cessation, before or during pregnancy improves birth weight, especially if the cessation occurs before 16 weeks of pregnancy.

C No evidence is documented that marijuana is a significant teratogen in humans. However, the presence of cannabinoid metabolites in the urine may identify patients who are likely to be concurrent users of other illicit substances. Adverse maternal effects of cocaine include profound vasoconstriction. Increasing evidence suggests that cocaine is a teratogen, especially during the first trimester. Opiate use has been associated with increased rates of stillbirth, IUGR, fetal and neonatal mortality, and prematurity. Like marijuana, opiates are not known to be teratogenic. Treatment with methadone is associated with improved pregnancy outcomes. Smoking has been identified as the leading preventable cause of low birth weight. Alcohol is the most common substance abused during pregnancy.

4. Which of the following statements about maternal screening is false?

A. First trimester screening is at least as good as second trimester screening for Down's syndrome and open NTD detection.

B. Average values for women carrying a fetus with Down's syndrome are low maternal serum alpha-fetoprotein (AFP), elevated human chorionic gonadotropin (hCG), low unconjugated estriol (uE3), and elevated dimeric inhibin A (DIA).

C. A typical profile for fetal trisomy 18 (Edward's syndrome) shows low AFP, very low hCG, and low uE3.

D. Elevated AFP levels are usually found in maternal serum (80% of cases) and amniotic fluid (>95% of cases) with open NTDs (>2.5 MoM).

E. First- and second-trimester screening may be offered to patients who decline invasive testing based upon advanced maternal age alone.

A First-trimester screening is performed between 11 and 14 weeks and includes maternal age, nuchal translucency, maternal serum free beta human chorionic gonadotropin (free β-hCG), and pregnancy-associated plasma protein-A (PAPP-A). It is at least as good as second-trimester screening for Down's syndrome, but it does not screen for open NTDs. Second-trimester screening is performed between 15 and 20 weeks and quantifies maternal serum AFP, hCG, uE3, and DIA, combined with maternal age.

5. All of the following are *true* about dating a pregnancy, *except:*

A. The 40-week gestational period is based on menstrual weeks rather than conception. This assumes that ovulation occurs during day 14 of a 28-day cycle.

B. Ultrasonographic dating is most accurate between 15 and 20 weeks of gestation because fetal structures are larger, allowing for more accurate measures.

C. In general, at 22 weeks' gestational age by LMP, if ultrasound measurements differ from LMP by more than 2 weeks, ultrasound dating is used.

D. A primigravid woman typically begins to feel the baby moving at around 19 weeks.

B Ultrasound dating is most accurate when performed at 7 to 11⅚ weeks of pregnancy. If LMP dating is consistent with ultrasonographic dating within the established range of accuracy for ultrasonography (see Table 4.4 in text), the estimated date of delivery is based on LMP. Choice D is also correct. In subsequent pregnancies, "quickening" is usually noted approximately 2 weeks earlier.

5

Normal Labor and Delivery, Operative Delivery, and Malpresentations

Valerie Jones

Read the following vignette to answer questions 1 and 2:

A 26-year-old gravida 2 para 1001 arrives to labor and delivery at 41 weeks' gestational age for induction of labor. Her cervical exam demonstrates a cervix that is 1 cm dilated, firm, anterior, 50% effaced, and −2 station. She is given a cervical ripening agent and placed on fetal monitoring and tocodynamometer.

1. This patient has a Bishop score of

A. 4

B. 5

C. 8

D. Cannot be determined

B Five. The Bishop score is calculated by using the three main components of a complete cervical exam: dilation (diameter of internal os), effacement (shortening and thinning of cervix as a percentage), and station (descent of presenting fetal part). In addition, the consistency and position of the cervix are factored into the Bishop score when determining the likelihood of successful labor induction (see Table 5.1). When the Bishop score exceeds 8, the likelihood of vaginal delivery after induction is similar to spontaneous labor. If there is a low Bishop score, cervical ripening with pharmacologic method may be indicated.

2. A few hours into the labor induction, the fetal monitoring shows a late deceleration after several episodes of frequent contractions. The most likely explanation for the deceleration is:

A. Maternal position on left lateral side

B. Uterine hyperstimulation from cervical ripening agent

C. Compression of the fetal head mediated by vagus nerve

B The late deceleration in this situation following episodes of contractions is most likely from uterine hyperstimulation, which can cause uteroplacental insufficiency and fetal hypoxia. Uterine hyperstimulation is a potential side effect with the use of prostaglandins. Choice A, Maternal position on left lateral side, is *not* correct because it is the ideal position for improving uterine blood flow and the vena caval compression from gravid uterus is relieved with this positioning. Finally, choice C is not correct because vagus nerve mediated response to fetal head compression is an example of an *early* deceleration.

3. A 25-year-old gravida 3 para 1102 at 35 weeks' gestational age is in the second stage of labor and has been pushing for 2 hours and is at +2 station. Maternal exhaustion has ensued and you are concerned about fetal distress. Which of the following is the most appropriate device to facilitate a safe delivery in this situation?

A. Low forceps

B. Soft cup vacuum

C. Mid forceps

D. Piper forceps

A Low forceps are an acceptable choice in this situation because the station is +2 or greater. Choice B is incorrect because vacuum use would be avoided in fetuses fewer than 36 weeks' estimated gestational age or with known thrombocytopenia due to increased risk of intracranial hemorrhage. Choice C is incorrect because mid forceps are more dangerous to apply than low forceps and refer to the situation in which the head is engaged but above the level of +2 station. Finally, choice D is incorrect because Piper forceps are used in breech deliveries only. Although sometimes helpful in expediting delivery, forceps have many known maternal complications, including uterine, cervical, or vaginal lacerations, bladder and ureteral injuries, and hematomas. Possible complications to the fetus are also present.

Read the following vignette to answer questions 4 and 5:

A 34-year-old gravida 4 para 2013 at 38 weeks' gestational age, with no prenatal care, presents to Labor and Delivery fully dilated with delivery appearing imminent. Cervical exam as well as ultrasound document complete breech position of fetus.

4. Correct maneuvering for breech delivery is as follows:

   A. Pinard's maneuver to deliver legs, rotate fetus sacrum anterior, wrap trunk in towel, delivery of arms when scapula visualized, then downward pressure on maxillary ridge to deliver head

   B. Pinard's maneuver to deliver legs, rotate fetus sacrum anterior, wrap trunk in towel, delivery of arms when scapula visualized, then downward pressure on mandible to deliver head

   C. Pinard's maneuver to deliver legs, rotate fetus sacrum posterior, wrap trunk in towel, delivery of arms when scapula visualized, then downward pressure on mandible to deliver head.

   A Choice A describes the correct sequence of events in the vaginal breech delivery. The Pinard maneuver includes medially placing fingers to each thigh and pressing out laterally to deliver legs (see Figure 5.7). Then the fetus is rotated to sacrum anterior and the trunk is wrapped in towel. When scapulas appear, place fingers over shoulders from back and rotate each arm from around the back. The humerus is followed down and each arm rotated across chest and out (Lovset's maneuver)(see Figure 5.8). Finally, the Mauriceau-Smellie-Veit maneuver is used by placing downward traction and pressure on maxillary ridge to deliver the head (see Figure 5.9).

5. Risk of breech delivery includes spinal cord injury if deflexion is present, birth trauma, cord prolapse, and head entrapment. Which of the following is an effective method of relieving head entrapment?

   A. Wood's corkscrew

   B. Rubin's maneuver

   C. Leopold's maneuver

   D. Dührssen's incisions on the cervix

D Dührssen's incisions made at the 2 o'clock, 6 o'clock, and 10 o'clock positions on the cervix can relieve head entrapment during breech delivery. However, care must be taken to avoid cervical vessels at 3 o'clock and 9 o'clock, which can cause hemorrhage. Choice A, Wood's corkscrew, is incorrect because it refers to a maneuver to relieve a shoulder dystocia in which the posterior shoulder is rotated 180 degrees forward in an attempt to deliver it first. Choice B, Rubin's maneuver, is another shoulder dystocia maneuver in which a hand is placed in the vagina behind fetal occiput and anterior shoulder is pushed obliquely. Finally, Choice C, Leopold's maneuver is incorrect because it refers to a series of four abdominal palpations of the gravid uterus to ascertain fetal lie, presentation, and estimated fetal weight.

6

Fetal Assessment

David Chang and Karin Blakemore

1. A 33-year-old gravida 2 para 1001 at 32 weeks' gestation presents to labor and delivery complaining about not feeling her baby move as it had previously. Her past medical history is remarkable for recently diagnosed chronic hypertension, diabetes, and tobacco use. Her blood pressure has been well controlled on the antihypertensive medications she is on. She is worried about the pregnancy's outcome because she was not hypertensive with her previous pregnancy. You put the baby on the monitor. What findings make the strip reassuring?

   A. One or more accelerations in 1 hour

   B. Two or more accelerations in 20 minutes

   C. Four or more decelerations in 20 minutes

   D. One acceleration in 1 hour

   B The nonstress test (NST) is one of the most frequently used modalities of antepartum testing. The NST is considered reactive if there are two fetal heart rate accelerations lasting 15 seconds and to 15 bpm above the baseline in a 20-minute period. Sometimes an extra 20 minutes of monitoring is done to account for the possibility of the fetus being in a sleep cycle. Vibroacoustic stimulation has also been used to increase the sensitivity of the NST.

2. Starting at what gestational age is the NST expected to be reactive?

   A. 20 weeks

   B. 16 weeks

C. 32 weeks

D. 10 weeks

> **C** The generation of fetal heart rate (FHR) patterns requires intact electrical conduction pathways, adequate myocardial neurohormone receptors, sympathetic and parasympathetic reflex arcs, and inherent myocardial contractility. In preterm pregnancies (24 to 32 weeks' gestational age), maturation of FHR central regulatory centers is incomplete. NSTs in this age group have lower mean amplitude (10 bpm) accelerations and brief spontaneous decelerations associated with movement. Quiet sleep states are also more common; longer observation may be needed to register sufficient acceleration counts. In general, testing is started at 32 weeks or after, the time when approximately 98% of NSTs are expected to be reactive.

3. The patient's NST is nonreactive after 40 minutes. You decide to perform a biophysical profile. Which of the following parameters is not included in this test?

A. Fetal breathing

B. Fetal tone

C. Fetal movement

D. Amniotic Fluid

E. Abdominal circumference

> **E** The biophysical profile is another test used to assess fetal well-being. In addition to the NST, the BPP uses four sonographic parameters: amniotic fluid volume, fetal tone, fetal body movements, and fetal breathing movements.
>
> The fetal biophysical profile score, when normal (8/10), is a direct, reliable, and accurate measure of normal tissue oxygenation and, by inference, absent central acidemia.

4. The patient delivered her baby after being induced secondary to severe pre-eclampsia at 35 weeks. She asks you if anything could be done next time she becomes pregnant to monitor the baby due to her multiple medical issues. You recommend:

A. Daily NSTs starting at 35 weeks

B. Biophysical profile every week starting at 20 weeks

C. Weekly NST starting at 28 weeks

D. Daily biophysical profile starting at 30 weeks

C The right time to start antepartum testing depends on several considerations, including severity of maternal disease, the risk of fetal death, prognosis of the neonate, and the risk of delivering prematurely from a false-positive test result. In pregnancies with multiple or worrisome conditions, testing may be started as early as 26 to 28 weeks. Several factors, including clinical judgment, should determine the frequency of testing. Any worsening of maternal condition or decrease in fetal activity should prompt fetal re-evaluation regardless of time elapsed since the last test.

5. A contraction stress test (CST) is considered positive if late decelerations occur in:

A. 50% or more of the contractions

B. All of the contractions

C. 25% or more of the contractions

D. One out of three contractions

A Contraction stress testing is used to assess fetal tolerance to contractions. Late decelerations with the ordinary hypoxemic stress of uterine contractions are a manifestation of a fetus that is beginning to develop marginal basal oxygenation. The fetus with a reserve of uteroplacental function will not display late decelerations. The test can be performed by use of intravenous oxytocin but can also be performed with nipple stimulation. A contraction stress test is positive if late decelerations follow 50% or more of contractions.

6. Which of the following is not a relative contraindication to perform a CST?

A. Preterm labor

B. Preterm premature rupture of membranes

C. Placenta previa

D. High risk for uterine rupture

E. Multiple pregnancy

E Relative contraindications to the CST usually include conditions that are associated with an increased risk of preterm labor and delivery, uterine rupture, or uterine bleeding. These conditions include preterm rupture of membranes, placenta previa, and high risk for uterine rupture.

7

Complications of Labor and Delivery

Matthew Guile

1. After a prolonged induction and maternal temperature of 38.6 during the second stage of labor, a 26-year-old P2002 is noted to be bleeding briskly soon after the placenta is expelled. Appropriate measures are taken to control the blood loss. What is the most likely cause of the patient's postpartum hemorrhage?

A. Retained products of conception

B. Uterine atony

C. Cervical laceration

D. Vaginal laceration

E. Consumptive coagulopathy

B Uterine atony is the number one cause of postpartum hemorrhage (PPH) and the leading cause of maternal death worldwide. It represents a failure of the normal physiologic process that halts postpartum blood loss. The uterus receives up to 600 mL/min of blood flow at term, which represents 10% of cardiac output.

Risk factors for PPH include overdistention of the uterus (e.g., polyhydramnios, macrosomia), prolonged or precipitous labor, and intrapartum infection. Assuming that adequate IV access exists, management of uterine atony begins with bimanual uterine massage. Bimanual massage and evacuation of clot from the lower uterine segment are the most effective treatments of uterine atony. Continued atony is approached in a stepwise fashion. Uterotonics are administered (Table 7.1) after ensuring that the patient has no medical contraindications to the pharmacologic agents. Further hemorrhage calls for

TABLE 7.1

Uterotonic Agents

Agent	Dosage	Comments/Relative Contraindications
Oxytocin (*Pitocin*)	10–40 U/L IV infusion of 10 mL/min; 10–40 U IM	Do not give IV push. With very high doses, can get antidiuretic effect with volume overload.
Methylergonovine maleate (*Methergine*)	0.2 mg IM every 2–4 hr. May give additional doses of 0.2 mg PO every 6 hr. Do not start PO until at least 4 hours after the last IM or IV dose.	Do not give to patients with pre-eclampsia, hypertension, or Raynaud's phenomenon. May cause nausea and vomiting.
15S-methyl prostaglandin $F_{2\alpha}$ analogs [Carboprost Tromethamine (*Hemabate*)]	0.25 mg IM (skeletal or myometrium) every 15–90 min to a maximum of 8 doses	Do not give to patients with asthma; significant renal, hepatic, or cardiac disease. May cause nausea, vomiting, diarrhea, pyrexia.
Prostaglandin E1 analog [Misoprostol (*Cytotec*)]	600–800 mcg PR	Caution in renal disease, cardiac disease.

From American College of Obstetricians and Gynecologists. Postpartum hemorrhage. ACOG Technical Bulletin No. 243. *Int J Gynaecol Obstet* 1998;61:79–86, with permission; Mousa HA, Alfirevic Z. Treatment for primary postpartum hemorrhage. *Cochrane Database Syst Rev* 2003;1, with permission; and You WB, Zahn CM. Postpartum hemorrhage: abnormally adherent placenta, uterine inversion, and puerperal hematomas. *Clin Obstet Gynecol* 2006;49:184–197, with permission.

increasingly invasive procedures, such as uterine tamponade with packing or balloon catheter, uterine artery embolization, and surgical intervention.

Other causes of PPH include laceration, retained products of conception, and coagulopathy. Most lacerations can be detected in the immediate postpartum period through careful inspection of the cervix, vagina, and rectum. Hemostasis is achieved through surgical repair. Retained products of conception should be suspected after a prolonged third stage of labor or in instances of abnormal placental vasculature. A final cause of PPH is consumptive coagulopathy. Surgical intervention is not indicated in this instance. Treatment is mainly supportive, consisting of early, judicious replenishment of volume and blood products.

2. A 31-year-old gravida 2 Para 0010 at term is admitted in active labor. The fetal heart tracing (FHT) has a baseline in the 130 to 140 range, moderate variability, and is reactive. Amniotomy is performed revealing moderate meconium staining of the amniotic fluid. Assuming that the FHT remains reactive, management should consist of which of the following?

A. Amnioinfusion

B. DeLee's suctioning of the infant on the perineum

C. Bulb suction and tactile stimulation on the perineum

D. Arrange for emergent intubation of the infant

E. Proceed with cesarean section

C Bulb suction and tactile stimulation on the perineum. Meconium is passed by the fetus while in utero in up to 20% of all live births. The association between meconium passage in utero and fetal indicators of hypoxia has led to the perception that meconium passage is indicative of fetal stress. Meconium aspiration syndrome is a life-threatening chemical pneumonitis that complicates 2% to 9% of these deliveries. Two traditional practices that were thought to decrease the risk of meconium aspiration, amnioinfusion and DeLee's suctioning of the nasopharynx and oropharynx, have recently been called into question. A multicenter randomized controlled trial showed no decrease in morbidity or mortality and, specifically, no decrease in meconium aspiration syndrome with amnioinfusion (4). A separate randomized controlled trial was designed to assess the effectiveness of DeLee's suctioning on the perineum. This study did not support the claim of decreased morbidity with this technique. Thus, neither amnioinfusion nor DeLee's suctioning on the perineum are indicated for vigorous term neonates with good respiratory effort. The American Association of Pediatrics 2005 guidelines for neonatal resuscitation recommend no endotracheal suctioning for vigorous, term neonates with meconium-stained amniotic fluid of any consistency (5). No reason exists to anticipate the need for either endotracheal intubation or cesarean section in this scenario.

3. An 18-year-old nulliparous patient presents to Labor and Delivery with spontaneous rupture of membranes at term; she states that her water broke approximately 3 hours earlier. Internal monitors are placed and the patient becomes febrile during the prolonged second stage of labor. Which of the following signs or would you expect on physical examination?

A. Shortness of breath

B. Suprapubic tenderness

C. Nausea and vomiting

D. Fundal tenderness

D Fundal tenderness. This patient most likely has chorioamnionitis. This infection of the fetal membranes and placenta often manifests as maternal and fetal tachycardia followed by fever. Other signs are uterine tenderness and the presence of malodorous amniotic fluid. The infection is polymicrobial, with the most common pathogens consisting of vaginal flora, such as ureaplasma urealyticum, group B streptococcus, and Gardnerella vaginalis. Lab work may reveal a leukocytosis with a left shift.

Risk factors present in this patient include nulliparity, prolonged rupture of membranes, and internal monitoring. The incidence of chorioamnionitis can be lessened by limiting the number of vaginal exams performed during labor.

Treatment consists of ampicillin and gentamicin during labor. The gentamicin is dosed every 8 hours. After a spontaneous vaginal delivery, the antibiotics are discontinued because the source of the infection has been removed. Antibiotic therapy is continued with the addition of anaerobic coverage after cesarean section.

4. The patient in question 3 delivers a liveborn male infant with Apgars of 8 and 9 at 1 and 5 minutes, respectively. On postpartum day 1, the patient is noted to have fundal tenderness and a temperature of 38.6°C. She denies rigors, chills, nausea, and vomiting. What is the proper management at this time?

A. CBC and blood cultures

B. Antipyretics and endometrial sampling for culture

C. Resumption of ampicillin and gentamicin

D. Initiation of triple antibiotic coverage with ampicillin, gentamicin, and clindamycin

E. Dilation and curettage for suspected retained products of conception

D Initiation of triple antibiotic coverage with ampicillin, gentamicin, and clindamycin. This patient has developed endometritis. The pathogenesis of endometritis is similar to chorioamnionitis: a polymicrobial infection of the endometrium and/or decidua with both gram-negative and gram-positive bacteria. The diagnosis of endometritis is primarily clinical, and, in this case, is strongly suggested by the patient's history of chorioamnionitis, fever, and fundal tenderness. Fever and fundal tenderness in the postpartum period are the hallmarks of endometritis.

Blood cultures are not indicated for endometritis in the absence of signs or symptoms of sepsis. Likewise, endometrial cultures are not helpful for management, because they will reveal polymicrobial colonization and infection. Although retained products of conception can result in fever and infection, a more likely presentation in the early postpartum period is continued cramping, bleeding, and uterine bogginess.

Treatment of endometritis consists of ampicillin, gentamicin, and clindamycin. The gentamicin is dosed daily in the postpartum period and is recommended that trough levels not be followed. The natural history of endometritis is such that the patient typically improves within 24 to 48 hours, as evidenced by decreased fundal tenderness and downtrending fever curve. Antibiotics are continued until the patient is afebrile for 24 to 48 hours.

5. A 33-year-old P2103 status-post lower segment transverse cesarean section had a postoperative course complicated by presumed endometritis. Appropriate antibiotics were initiated on postoperative day (POD) 1. The patient's temperature curve is notable for daily spiking fevers that have continued until POD 5, despite antibiotic administration. Complete physical exam is only notable for tachycardia and no fundal tenderness. Pelvic exam is within normal limits. The incision is clean, dry, and intact. What is the likely cause of the patient's fever?

A. Pneumonia

B. Atelectasis

C. Urinary tract infection

D. Septic pelvic thrombophlebitis

E. Pelvic abscess

D Septic pelvic thrombophlebitis. This patient has a clinical presentation consistent with septic pelvic thrombophlebitis, which is a diagnosis of exclusion. The failure of the patient's fever to respond to triple antibiotic therapy, and the spiking pattern, are both suggestive of this diagnosis. A pelvic abscess would likely reveal a more dramatic physical exam, and a pulmonary etiology is unlikely in this patient.

Septic pelvic thrombophlebitis complicates 1/200 to 1/3,000 deliveries, with cesarean delivery being a common antecedent. The venous channels involved are the deep pelvic or ovarian veins, which are dramatically engorged during pregnancy. Virchow's triad of hypercoagulability, stasis and vessel injury can be present during the late antepartum and early postpartum period, predisposing the patient to thrombi. The consensus is that the spiking pattern of the fevers is due to daily showers of microemboli that can travel through the inferior vena cava to the pulmonary bed.

Diagnostic workup involves thorough pelvic exam, chest and abdominal radiographs, and CT scan of the abdomen and pelvis. The positive predictive value of imaging is excellent, but negative studies do not exclude the diagnosis.

Treatment should be initiated for septic pelvic thrombophlebitis after the complete workup reveals no other source of fevers. The ampicillin, gentamicin, and clindamycin should be continued, with the addition of intravenous heparin. The fevers should resolve within 1 to 5 days, thus confirming the diagnosis. The optimal length of heparin therapy is controversial, with expert opinion ranging from 1 to 14 days after fever resolution.

References

1. American College of Obstetricians and Gynecologists. Postpartum hemorrhage. ACOG Technical Bulletin No. 243. *Int J Gynaecol Obstet* 1998;61:79–86.
2. Mousa HA, Alfirevic Z. Treatment for primary postpartum hemorrhage. *Cochrane Database Syst Rev* 2003;1.
3. You WB, Zahn CM. Postpartum hemorrhage: abnormally adherent placenta, uterine inversion, and puerperal hematomas. *Clin Obstet Gynecol* 2006;49:184–197.

4. Fraser WD, Hofmeyr J, Lede R, et al for the Amnioinfusion Trial Group. Amnioinfusion for the prevention of the meconium aspiration syndrome. *N Engl J Med* 2005;353:909–917.

5. American Heart Association, American Academy of Pediatrics. 2005 American Heart Association (AHA) Guidelines for Cardiopulmonary Resuscitation (CPR) and Emergency Cardiovascular Care (ECC) of Pediatric and Neonatal Patients: Neonatal Resuscitation Guidelines. *Pediatrics* 2006;117:1029–1038.

8

Gestational Complications

Kimberly B. Fortner

1. A 24-year-old gravida 1 P0 at 30 weeks' gestational age comes to the office complaining of significant shortness of breath and increased abdominal girth. This prenatal visit is only her second visit, with the first being at 7 weeks, confirming gestational age. On examination, her fundal height is 37 cm. All of the following could be linked to her diagnosis, *except:*

A. Fetal esophageal atresia

B. Fetal renal agenesis

C. Fetal trisomy 21

D. Maternal diabetes

E. Congenital cytomegalovirus infection

> **B** Fetal renal agenesis. The patient has poor prenatal care but seems to have appropriate dating, as evidenced by her initial visit at 7 weeks. The patient most likely has a diagnosis of polyhydramnios. True evaluation of polyhydramnios is by sonographic measurement of amniotic fluid volume (more than 2,000 mL at any gestational age, more than the 95th percentile for gestational age, or an AFI greater than 25 cm at term). The majority of cases are idiopathic. However, other causes of increased fetal urine production, increased fetal transudation of fluid across exposed surfaces, impaired swallowing, or impaired absorption of the amniotic fluid should be ruled out. Such causes include fetal chromosomal anomalies or structural malformations leading to decreased absorption or increased production (esophageal atresia or bowel obstruction). Renal agenesis may lead to decreased production and resultant oligohy-

dramnios. Additional causes for polyhydramnios include diabetes, isoimmunization, and congenital infections.

The following scenario applies to questions 2 and 3:

2. A 27-year-old gravida 5 P 3103 comes for her registration visit at 32 weeks by the first day of her LMP. Her history reveals previous diagnosis of fetal demise in utero at 34 weeks. She reports a history of polysubstance abuse, including cocaine and previous diagnosis of hypertension. Currently, her fetal tracing is reassuring.

On assessment, her fundal height is measuring 28 cm. Assuming her gestational age is correct, your management includes:

A. Admission to Labor and Delivery

B. Pelvic exam to rule out rupture of membranes and then evaluation of fetal growth

C. Obtain NST and send her home with instructions for kick counts

D. Obtain sonogram for growth and follow-up in 1 week

> **B** Pelvic exam to rule out rupture of membranes and then evaluation of fetal growth. The patient is measuring less than suggested dates. Her smaller size could be a result of growth restriction, incorrect dating, or low fluid. After excluding dating as the cause, the patient must be evaluated for oligohydramnios and growth restriction. The clinical conditions commonly leading to oligohydramnios are ruptured membranes, fetal urinary tract malformations, postdates pregnancy, and placental insufficiency. Rupture of membranes must be considered at any gestational age. No current indications for delivery are present.

3. On sonogram, the patient is found to have normal amniotic fluid index, but sonographic measurements of the abdomen are consistent with 28 weeks, femur length is consistent with 29 weeks, and head measurements are in agreement with 32 weeks. Workup for this patient should include all of the following, *except:*

A. Nutritional assessment

B. Evaluation for hypercoagulable disorders

C. Workup to rule out pre-eclampsia

D. Evaluation of maternal and paternal birth weights

E. Evaluation for fetal chromosomes and infectious studies

D Evaluation of maternal and paternal birth weights. Though 70% of intrauterine growth restriction (IUGR) cases are constitutionally small, likely due to maternal and paternal stature, the case is probably not the same here, and a workup should first exclude other causes. This case describes a diagnosis of asymmetric IUGR. The remaining plans all include evaluation for causes of asymmetric growth restriction.

4. A 30-year-old gravida 1 P0 at 12 weeks with a twin pregnancy comes to the office for her first prenatal visit since being diagnosed with twins. The patient has been reading on the Internet and wants to know if her twins cleaved on day 5. You explain she is probably correct because her twins are

A. Dichorionic/diamniotic, dizygotic twins

B. Dichorionic/diamniotic, monozygotic twins

C. Monochorionic/diamniotic, monozygotic twins

D. Monochorionic/monoamniotic, monozygotic twins

E. Conjoined twins

C Monochorionic/diamniotic, monozygotic twins. **Dichorionic/diamniotic** and **dizygotic twins** are a product of fertilization of multiple ova. Each fetus has its own placenta and each fetus is contained within a complete amniotic-chorionic membrane. **Dichorionic/diamniotic monozygotic twins** occur if cleavage occurs in the first 3 days after fertilization. The twins will have separate amnions and chorions, as in dizygotic twins. **Monochorionic/diamniotic monozygotic twins** occur between the fourth and eighth days after fertilization. The twins will share a single placenta because the chorionic layer has already formed. However, they still have separate amniotic sacs. **Monochorionic/monoamniotic monozygotic twins** develop if cleavage occurs after the eighth day, and the twins share a single placenta and a single amniotic sac, because the amnion and chorion were formed before the embryos divided. Later cleavage results in conjoined twins and is even rarer.

9

Preterm Labor and Premature Rupture of Membranes

Alice Chung Cootauco and Janyne E. Althaus

1. A 30-year-old gravida 3 Para 0202 at 22 weeks' gestational age presents to the clinic for her routine obstetric care. Which of the following has been shown to reduce her incidence of having another preterm delivery?

   A. Oral terbutaline
   B. Terbutaline pump
   C. Medroxyprogesterone injections
   D. Magnesium sulfate
   E. Bed rest

   C Vaginal progesterone suppositories and medroxyprogesterone injections have been shown to reduce the incidence of preterm delivery in patients with a history of previous preterm delivery in randomized double-blind, placebo-controlled trials. The progesterone suppositories are administered daily, whereas the injections are weekly.

   No randomized control trial has shown efficacy of bed rest in preventing a preterm delivery. In fact, bed rest can cause greater morbidity with increased risk of deep vein thrombosis. Of importance for patients on bed rest is to have TEDs and/or SCDs and physical therapy to prevent DVT formation and maintain muscle strength.

   In patients with established preterm labor, tocolytics, such as intravenous magnesium sulfate and terbutaline, have been shown to help stop labor temporarily, on the average, for 72 hours. Randomized controlled trials that compare patients, successfully tocolyzed previously and then maintained on oral terbutaline versus no terbutaline, showed no difference in pregnancy outcome, including gestational age at delivery and neonatal outcome. Two randomized controlled studies compared patients, successfully tocolyzed, with and without continuous terbutaline pump. They both showed no difference in gestational age at delivery or neonatal outcome.

A randomized control trial that examined prevention of preterm delivery in high-risk patients with oral magnesium gluconate 1 g four times daily showed no difference in birth weight or gestational age at delivery. Of note, the randomized control trials that investigated the use of terbutaline, nifedipine, and bed rest included patients who were already in preterm labor and not necessarily women who had a history of preterm delivery receiving prophylactic treatment before showing signs of preterm labor.

2. Which of the following is/are contraindications to magnesium sulfate tocolysis?

A. Preterm premature rupture of membranes (PPROM)

B. Placental abruption

C. Chorioamnionitis

D. Myasthenia gravis

E. C and D

> **E** Magnesium sulfate is used for cessation of contractions in preterm labor or seizure prophylaxis in patients with pre-eclampsia. Myasthenia gravis is an autoimmune disorder in which IgG antibodies are present that destroy the acetylcholine receptors at the postsynaptic junction in striated muscle. Calcium ions are involved in activating contraction of muscle fibers. Magnesium is hypothesized to compete with calcium in this process, thereby decreasing muscle contractility. By exacerbating muscle weakness, magnesium sulfate should not be used in patients with myasthenia gravis. A case report exists of respiratory arrest in a patient with myasthenia gravis receiving magnesium tocolysis. Alternatives to magnesium sulfate prophylaxis, such as Dilantin, should be used in myasthenia gravis patients with pre-eclampsia.

Magnesium sulfate can be helpful in stabilizing a placental abruption. The bleeding in an abruption can irritate uterine muscle, causing contractions. These contractions can then make the abruption worse, resulting in further bleeding. By stopping the contractions, the cycle can be stopped. If there is fetal tachycardia or late decelerations, the mother has signs of worsening anemia with hypotension and tachycardia, or the bleeding is significant, the fetus should be delivered.

Patients with chorioamnionitis should be delivered regardless of gestational age because the fetus no longer benefits from being in utero. Ampicillin and gentamicin should be started and labor should be induced or cesarean section performed, depending on the fetal presentation, cervical exam, and fetal tracing.

PPROM after 34 weeks should not be tocolyzed secondary to risk of infection and no difference in neonatal outcome. Between 24 and 32 weeks, antenatal steroids can be administered to promote fetal lung maturity. If the patient is contracting after initial rupture of membranes, and the fetal heart tracing is stable and no evidence of chorioamnionitis is present, then magnesium sulfate tocolysis can be administered to allow optimal timing of steroids for fetal lung maturity.

3. A 24-year-old gravida 1 Para 0 at 35 weeks' gestational age presents to Labor and Delivery with regular contractions. No evidence of rupture of membranes and fetal heart tracing is reactive. Tocodynamometer shows contractions every 2 to 3 minutes. Cervix is 5 cm dilated and 100% effaced. Group B streptococcus status is unknown. She reports having a rash and itching with penicillin. What is the next step of management?

A. Intravenous magnesium sulfate

B. Oral Indocin

C. Betamethasone

D. Cefazolin

E. Clindamycin

D Group B streptococcus (GBS) can cause morbidity and mortality to newborn infants—a gram-positive organism that is commonly colonized in pregnant women in the urinary tract, vagina, and rectum. Invasive GBS infections in

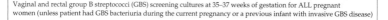

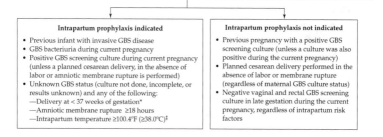

Vaginal and rectal group B streptococci (GBS) screening cultures at 35–37 weeks of gestation for ALL pregnant women (unless patient had GBS bacteriuria during the current pregnancy or a previous infant with invasive GBS disease)

Intrapartum prophylaxis indicated	**Intrapartum prophylaxis not indicated**

• Previous infant with invasive GBS disease
• GBS bacteriuria during current pregnancy
• Positive GBS screening culture during current pregnancy (unless a planned cesarean delivery, in the absence of labor or amniotic membrane rupture is performed)
• Unknown GBS status (culture not done, incomplete, or results unknown) and any of the following:
  —Delivery at < 37 weeks of gestation*
  —Amniotic membrane rupture ≥18 hours
  —Intrapartum temperature ≥100.4°F (≥38.0°C)‡
	• Previous pregnancy with a positive GBS screening culture (unless a culture was also positive during the current pregnancy)
	• Planned cesarean delivery performed in the absence of labor or membrane rupture (regardless of maternal GBS culture status)
	• Negative vaginal and rectal GBS screening culture in late gestation during the current pregnancy, regardless of intrapartum risk factors

Figure 9.1. Indications for intrapartum antibiotic prophylaxis to prevent perinatal GBS disease.

newborns can cause sepsis, pneumonia, or meningitis. In 2002, the Centers for Disease Control and Prevention revised guidelines for prevention of perinatal GBS disease. See the diagram for indications for intrapartum prophylaxis. When a patient has a penicillin allergy, the GBS culture must be labeled as such so that the lab will check for sensitivities to clindamycin and erythromycin.

The Centers for Disease Control and Prevention also released recommended regimens for intrapartum antimicrobial prophylaxis for perinatal GBS disease prevention. See Figure 9.2 for the appropriate antibiotic for a patient requiring GBS prophylaxis.

Recommended	Penicillin G, 5 million units IV initial dose, then 2.5 million units IV every 4 hours until delivery
Alternative	Ampicillin, 2 g IV initial dose, then 1 g IV every 4 hours until delivery
If penicillin allergic Patients not at high risk for anaphylaxis	Cefazolin, 2 g IV initial dose, then 1 g IV every 8 hours until delivery

Patients at high risk for anaphylaxis
  GBS susceptible to clindamycin and erythromycin
	Clindamycin, 900 mg IV every 8 hours until delivery
	             OR
	Erythromycin, 500 mg IV every 6 hours until delivery

GBS resistant to clindamycin or erythromycin or susceptibility unknown	Vancomycin, 1 g IV every 12 hours until delivery

Figure 9.2. Recommended regimens for intrapartum antimicrobial prophylaxis for perinatal GBS disease prevention.

4. The advent of tocolytics, antibiotic regimens, and corticosteroids has decreased the incidence of preterm delivery. Is this statement *true* or *false?*

> **FALSE** The incidence of preterm delivery has not changed. The incidence has remained between 9% and 11%. Unexplained differences exist in the rate of preterm delivery among races. The increasing use of assisted reproduction has also contributed to greater numbers of multiple gestation pregnancies which are associated with preterm labor.

5. A 29-year-old gravida 2 para 0010 at 29 weeks' gestational age, with PPROM, complains of contractions. She is status post betamethasone times two doses and is on her fourth day of antibiotics. She is afebrile, fetal heart rate is in 170s, and abdominal exam reveals fundal tenderness. Tocodynamometer shows contractions every 8 to 10 minutes. Her cervix is visually 4 cm, which is changed from the previous exam. Ultrasound confirms vertex presentation. Your next step of management is:

A. Subcutaneous terbutaline sulfate

B. Intravenous magnesium sulfate

C. Pitocin augmentation

D. Continue amoxicillin and erythromycin

E. Cesarean section

> **C** The incidence of chorioamnionitis in PPROM is 15% to 25%. An increased incidence of neonatal sepsis exists with PPROM. Despite this patient remaining afebrile, her physical exam shows evidence of infection with fundal tenderness and fetal tachycardia. Once there is evidence of chorioamnionitis or any sign of compromise to the fetus, delivery should be performed. Because the fetus's presentation is vertex, the next step should be induction of labor with Pitocin. GBS prophylaxis should be given, as determined by her GBS culture result.

10

Third Trimester Bleeding

Nancy Arquette and Cynthia J. Holcroft

1. Placental abruption is associated with all of the following risk factors, *except:*

A. Hypertension

B. Advanced maternal age

C. Multiple gestation

D. Tobacco use

E. All of the above

> **E** Placental abruption is associated with all of the above risk factors. Other factors include cocaine use, chorioamnionitis, abdominal trauma, placental implantation over myomas, polyhydramnios with an overdistended uterus, external cephalic version, and inherited thrombophilias. It is also important to remember that placental abruption may occur in the setting of no associated risk factors.

2. A 24-year-old G3P2002 at 36 2/7 weeks' gestation presents to Labor and Delivery triage with a complaint of vaginal bleeding. It began approximately 3 hours ago, and she has used about five sanitary napkins since it began. She reports mild-to-moderate abdominal pain, no gush of clear fluid, and decreased fetal movement. She has no history of placental abnormalities. Which of the following is most likely to help establish a presumed diagnosis of placental abruption?

A. Ultrasound

B. Apt test

C. Continued or increased vaginal bleeding

D. Maternal CBC

C Although the differential diagnosis of vaginal bleeding in the third trimester is somewhat broad, this patient presented with heavy vaginal bleeding and abdominal pain, two hallmark signs of placental abruption. From her history we know that she does not have placenta previa or vasa previa. Therefore, if we were concerned about placental abruption, increased vaginal bleeding would most likely make us think that the patient was having an abruption. She is already soaking over 1 pad per hour; if her bleeding became worse, we would consider a cesarean section in this patient and confirm abruption later. Ultrasound is most useful in diagnosing placenta previa and vasa previa, and it is less sensitive in diagnosing an abruption. However, ultrasound may show a hypoechoic area between the uterine wall and placenta in large abruptions. The Apt test is useful in determining whether vaginal blood is maternal or fetal in origin. A maternal CBC will tell us the hematocrit and platelets, which may help in determining the status of the mother. It may also help in determining the amount of blood loss and the need for transfusion; however, this method is not the most helpful in diagnosing an abruption.

3. Upon examining the patient in question 2, you find that her vital signs are stable, her abdominal exam is benign, no evidence of membrane rupture exists, no active bleeding is seen from the cervical os, and her cervix is 2 cm dilated and 70% effaced. The tocodynamometer shows contractions about every 7 minutes, and the fetal heart rate is in the 130s with moderate variability and no accelerations after an hour of continuous monitoring. The patient is moderately uncomfortable with her contractions and would like to know what your plan is. You decide to:

A. Admit her and induce her labor

B. Admit her and proceed with cesarean section

C. Have her ambulate for 2 hours, then re-examine with possible discharge home

D. Discharge home with labor warnings and bleeding precautions

E. Keep her for observation and continued monitoring

E In addition to presenting with signs concerning for a placental abruption (significant vaginal bleeding and abdominal pain), the fetal heart rate is not reactive, therefore observation and continued monitoring is warranted. Continue to monitor for other episodes of bleeding or pain, as well as a decline in fetal status. Because the fetal heart rate is not reactive, a biophysical profile and amniotic fluid index should be performed. During continued observation, you would also want to send labs on the patient, such as type and screen, CBC, and urine toxicology screen. At this point, nothing in her exam warrants induction of labor or immediate cesarean section. Mother and fetus are both currently stable without signs of active labor, and the fetus is still preterm. Ambulation is not a good choice in someone who had recent significant bleeding and a nonreactive fetal heart rate strip. For the reasons mentioned previously, immediate discharge in the patient is also not a good option.

4. Placenta previa is associated with all of the following factors, *except:*

A. Female>male gender fetus

B. Congenital malformations

C. Breech presentation

D. Preterm premature rupture of membranes

E. Intrauterine growth restriction

A Placenta previa is more often associated with the male gender. Choices B through E are all associated with placenta previa. Risk factors for placenta previa include previous cesarean section, multiparity, advanced maternal age, tobacco use, residing in higher altitudes, myomas, and previous uterine surgery, including dilation and curettage.

5. A 32-year-old G3P1011 at 32 weeks' gestation, with a known complete placenta previa, presents to Labor and Delivery triage for her second episode of vaginal bleeding. She has soaked two pads over the course of 4 hours and her bleeding has now stopped. She denies a gush of clear fluid or abdominal pain and reports good fetal movement. She received betamethasone on her first admission for vaginal bleeding approximately 3 weeks ago. She lives 45 minutes away, and her husband is out of town. She appears very unsettled and is worried about another bleeding episode. However, she wants to go home and is demanding to have a cesarean section in 4 days upon the return of her husband. All parts of the exam are within normal limits, she is seldom contracting, and the fetal heart rate is reassuring. Your next step is to:

A. Admit her for immediate cesarean section

B. Admit her for continued observation and reassurance

C. Discharge home now that it appears her bleeding has stopped

D. Discharge home as long as she promises to return for her cesarean section in 4 days

E. Readminister betamethasone and begin tocolytic therapy

B Admit her for continued observation and reassurance. The current recommendations are for each episode of bleeding with a complete previa, the patient should be admitted to the hospital for observation and expectant management. Mother and fetus are both hemodynamically stable and the fetus is preterm. Hospital management would include bed rest with bathroom privileges, fetal monitoring with testing as warranted, periodic assessment of maternal hematocrit, and active type and screen. Because the incident is her second episode of bleeding, if it stops for greater than 1 week, then she may be able to be discharged under the right conditions. Choice A is incorrect because no current indication is present for delivery, the fetus is preterm, and both mother and fetus are stable. Choices C and D are incorrect because hospital admission is mandatory for vaginal bleeding with a complete previa. Choice E is incorrect because the patient has already been given betamethasone for fetal lung maturity, and tocolysis is usually not warranted unless it is given along with administration of steroids.

11

Perinatal Infections

Amy Johnson and Brenda Ross

1. A 25-year-old G2P1001 at 38 weeks' gestation presents in active labor. A group B *Streptococcus* (GBS) culture performed at 36 weeks was noted to be positive. The patient reports a history of anaphylaxis to penicillin. However, GBS sensitivities were not sent. The appropriate management is:

   A. No antibiotic therapy unless rupture of membranes >18 hr
   B. Clindamycin 900 mg IV q 8 hr
   C. Cefazolin 2 g IV loading dose, then 1 g IV q 8 hr
   D. Vancomycin 1 g IV q 12 hr

   D Vancomycin. GBS vaginal colonization occurs in approximately 20% of women. Transmission to the fetus can occur as an ascending infection or with fetal passage during the labor process. Although the rate of transmission can range from 40% to 70%, rarely (only 1% to 2%) do full-term infants develop serious complications, such as sepsis, meningitis, or pneumonia. However, preterm infants are more susceptible to GBS infections. The 2002 Centers of Disease Control and Prevention (CDC) guidelines recommend universal screening between 35 and 37 weeks' gestation. Patients with a positive urine culture for GBS during the pregnancy, or a recent positive genital culture, or a previous infant with GBS sepsis should receive GBS prophylaxis (see Figs. 9.1 and 9.2).

2. A 32-year-old G0P0 at 9 weeks' gestation presents with fatigue, sore throat, and atypical lymphocytosis. A monospot is negative. Further workup should include:

A. Parvovirus IgM

B. Toxoplasmosis IgG and IgM

C. Hepatitis A

D. Rubella PCR

B Toxoplasmosis. Although the vast majority of patients with toxoplasmosis (approximately 90%) are asymptomatic, patients can present with a mononucleosis-like syndrome. Symptoms typically include fatigue, malaise, cervical lymphadenopathy, sore throat, and atypical lymphocytosis. Fetal infection occurs during the spreading phase of the parasitemia. The rate of fetal transmission increases with gestational age (15% in the first trimester, 30% in the second trimester, and 60% in the third trimester). The most common symptoms reported in neonates include low birth weight, hepatosplenomegaly, icterus, and anemia. In addition, late sequelae can occur, such as vision loss, hearing loss, and psychomotor and mental retardation. However, up to 90% of infants with congenital toxoplasmosis are initially asymptomatic at birth.

Screening for toxoplasmosis is not routine, because most women with acute toxoplasmosis are asymptomatic, and often the diagnosis is not suspected until an affected infant is born. Women who do present with symptoms of acute toxoplasmosis should be tested for both IgM and IgG titers. Table 11.1 directs interpretation of IgG and IgM results. Additional diagnostic tests include the Sabin-Feldman

TABLE 11.1

Interpretation of *Toxoplasma* Serology Results

IgM*	IgG	Interpretation
+	−	Possible acute infection; IgG titers should be reassessed in several weeks
+	+	Possible acute infection
−	+	Remote infection
−	−	Susceptible; uninfected

IgG, immunoglobulin G; IgM, immunoglobulin M; +, positive; −, negative.
*IgM titers may remain elevated for up to 1 year.

dye test, the indirect fluorescent antibody test, and ELISA. Fetal testing can be performed via amniocentesis for PCR. Common ultrasound findings include pericardial and pleural effusions, ventricular dilation, hepatosplenomegaly, and intrahepatic lesions.

Patients with parvovirus B19 typically present with symptoms of fifth disease. These symptoms include erythematous macular facial rash and acute joint swelling. Patients with hemolytic anemia, such as sickle cell disease, may develop aplastic anemia secondary to parvovirus.

Hepatitis A, which is primarily transmitted through fecal-oral contamination, usually occurs as an epidemic. Common symptoms include fatigue, anorexia, nausea, vomiting, and right upper quadrant abdominal pain. Patients typically have signs of jaundice, abdominal pain, and hepatomegaly. In rare cases, patients can develop fulminant coagulopathy and encephalopathy. Perinatal transmission of hepatitis A has not been documented. Diagnosis includes a full hepatitis screen. Positive hepatitis IgM antibodies indicate recent infection, whereas IgG antibodies will likely always remain positive after an infection.

In the United States, rubella vaccines are routinely given. However, approximately 20% of the population still remain susceptible to infection. Rubella is spread via nasopharyngeal droplets. The incubation period is anywhere from 2 to 3 weeks. Patients are most contagious 1 week before the onset of symptoms but remain infectious until 4 to 5 days after the onset of rash. As many as one third of patients with a rubella infection will not exhibit symptoms. Typically, the symptoms are mild and consist of a maculopapular rash lasting for several days. Other symptoms include lymphadenopathy (particularly postauricular and occipital), arthritis, fatigue, and headache. Unfortunately, 50% of fetuses are infected with rubella during the first trimester, a critical time period for organ development and are thus at risk for major congenital anomalies. The most common anomalies include congenital cataracts (10%), micro-ophthalmia, congenital heart anomalies (10% to 20%), and sensorineural deafness (60% to 75%). Other effects include mental retardation and microcephaly. Approximately 30% of infants are asymptomatic at birth but can develop late sequelae, including thyroid disorders, diabetes, and precocious puberty. Rubella infections are typically diagnosed through antibody testing. Patients should be tested at the time of exposure and then 2 weeks later. Note that some patients may take up to 4 weeks to test positive. Acute infection is indicated by a titer increase of fourfold or greater. If the patient has a positive antibody test at the time of exposure, then they are immune and no further testing is indicated. Prenatal diagnosis can be made if fetal blood tests positive for IgM.

3. A 29-year-old G2P1001 at 18 weeks' gestation presents with symptoms of joint pains and an erythematous rash on her face. She currently works in a day-care center. The most likely diagnosis is:

A. Varicella

B. Parvovirus

C. Herpes zoster

D. Rubeola

B Parvovirus. Patients with parvovirus B19 typically present with symptoms, including an erythematous macular facial rash and acute joint swelling. A history of hemolytic anemia, such as sickle cell disease, predisposes patients with parvovirus to the development of aplastic anemia. Any pregnant woman who is exposed to a child with fifth disease or presents with a purpuric rash should be tested for parvovirus by measuring IgG and IgM titers. The ideal time to draw titers is 10 days after the exposure. Parvovirus IgG is often detected by the seventh day of symptoms and remains positive for several years. In general, IgM appears within 3 days of symptoms, peaks in 30 to 60 days, and may persist for several months.

In patients who are immunocompromised and exposed to parvovirus, IV gamma globulin can be given as prophylaxis. In addition, women who develop aplastic anemia should be treated. The fetus should be monitored with serial ultrasounds, because fetal hydrops is a known complication. Hydrops typically develops within 6 to 10 weeks of maternal infection and often requires fetal intrauterine blood transfusion.

Varicella is an airborne pathogen, which typically occurs in outbreaks during the winter months. Fortunately, most women of childbearing age have already been exposed or have received the varicella vaccine, and therefore infection occurs less than 1 of every 1,000 pregnancies. However, when the infection does occur during pregnancy, it can be particularly dangerous. The virus has an incubation period of 10 to 21 weeks and is most infectious 1 to 2 days before onset of the pustular rash and persists until crusting has occurred. Diagnosis is made clinically, with a rash that typically starts on the head and spreads to the trunk and extremities. Pregnant women are at risk for developing varicella pneumonia, which should be managed aggressively with acyclovir, because of its high mortality rate.

Maternal infection that occurs within the first 20 weeks of gestation confers an increased risk of fetal congenital anomalies, which is estimated to be approximately 5%. Congenital varicella syndrome includes abnormalities, such as limb reduction anomalies, IUGR, retardation, chorioretinitis, microcephaly, and cutaneous scars.

If maternal varicella infection occurs within 5 days of delivery, the neonate is at significant risk for developing varicella. Neonatal disease carries a mortality rate as high as 30%. However, if delivery occurs after 5 days of maternal infection, the infant has likely received maternal antibodies, which will confer protection from the infection. Therefore, some experts recommend tocolysis and immunoglobulin, if labor occurs within 5 days of maternal infection.

Herpes zoster, also known as shingles, characteristically presents with a unilateral rash. The rash is vesicular and occurs along dermatomes. Herpes zoster infection is a reactivation of varicella, which is usually more prevalent in older and immunocompromised patients. It is important to note that zoster is neither more common nor more severe in pregnancy and is not associated with fetal sequelae.

Rubeola typically presents with prodromal symptoms of cough, coryza, conjunctivitis, and fever, which is followed by the onset of Koplik's spots and a maculopapular rash. Fortunately, most women in the United States have been vaccinated against rubeola because of its highly contagious nature and increased risks during pregnancy.

4. Maternal infection with rubeola is most often complicated by

A. Hemolysis

B. Pneumonia

C. Hepatitis

D. Cardiomyopathy

B Pneumonia. Rubeola presents with evolving symptoms and typically has an incubation period of 10 to 14 days. Patients initially present with 2 days of fever, conjunctivitis, cough, and coryza. Then on the second or third day, Koplik's spots (pinpoint gray-white spots surrounded by erythema) can appear followed by a maculopapular rash. Measles may be complicated by pneumonia, encephalitis, or otitis media. Rare complications include encephalitis and subacute sclerosing panencephalitis, both of which carry a high mortality rate. Measles are highly contagious and remain communicable from the onset of symptoms until 3 to 4 days after the appearance of the rash. In addition, the overall morbidity and mortality of measles is increased during pregnancy, because women are at a greater risk of pulmonary complications. Pregnant women with acute measles outbreak are at risk for preterm labor, dehydration, and bacterial pneumonia.

The diagnosis is made clinically. However, serologies can be obtained if the clinical picture is atypical. Universal screening for measles immunity is recommended as part of routine prenatal care. Nonimmune women should receive the vaccine postpartum but should be advised to use birth control for 3 months because the vaccine is a live attenuation. Nonimmune women who are exposed to measles should prophylactically receive immunoglobulin. If the woman develops symptoms of measles, treatment is limited to supportive care. Infants should receive immune globulin, if delivery occurs within 7 to 10 days of the mother developing measles.

Infants are at risk of infection secondary to transplacental transmission. Serial ultrasounds should be preformed to evaluate for fetal growth restriction, oligohydramnios, and microcephaly.

5. When counseling a patient with a primary CMV infection during pregnancy, the following information should be included:

A. 1% risk of fetal transmission, which can result in hearing loss, visual disturbances, learning disabilities, and mental retardation

B. 10% risk of fetal transmission, which can result in cutaneous scars, limb-reduction anomalies, malformed digits, muscle atrophy, and growth restriction

C. 40% risk of fetal transmission, which can result in hearing loss, visual disturbances, learning disabilities, and mental retardation

D. 80% risk of fetal transmission, which can result in cutaneous scars, limb-reduction anomalies, malformed digits, muscle atrophy, and growth restriction

C CMV infection is the most common congenital infection in the United States and has been reported to affect as many as 2% of neonates. Approximately half of the U.S. population is CMV seropositive and the virus can be spread via bodily fluids, including saliva, semen, cervical secretions, blood, urine, and breast milk. Therefore, transmission can occur from mother to child both in utero and postpartum. CMV is typically asymptomatic in the immunocompetent patient, presenting with symptoms in only 1% to 5% of patients. However, symptoms can include low-grade fever, malaise, arthralgia, and pharyngitis with lymphadenopathy. After a primary infection, CMV becomes latent. Mothers determined to be seronegative for CMV before conception, or early in the pregnancy, have a 1% to 4% risk of contracting CMV during pregnancy, with a 30% to 40% rate of fetal transmission. Fetal infection most commonly is the result of a recurrent maternal CMV infection. However, recurrent maternal CMV infections rarely lead to congenital anomalies in the fetus because partial protection is provided by maternal antibodies. Only 10% to 15% of infected infants have clinically apparent disease at birth, yet 90% of these will develop long-term sequelae. Of the remaining 85% to 90%, with asymptomatic infections at birth, only 5% to 15% will develop long-term sequelae. The risk of fetal sequelae is higher if the infection occurs earlier in the pregnancy. Common symptoms seen in the infected fetus include petechiae, hepatosplenomegaly, jaundice, microcephaly with periventricular calcifications, oligohydramnios, IUGR, chorioretinitis, and nonimmune hydrops. Unfortunately, congenital CMV infection can be fatal in as many as one third of affected neonates. Of the survivors, approximately 70% will develop hearing loss, visual loss, motor impairments, developmental disabilities, and mental retardation.

Unfortunately, maternal infection can be detected reliably only by documenting seroconversion of serial immunoglobulin G (IgG) measurements. Intrauterine detection of fetal infection can be detected via serial ultrasounds as well as amniocentesis for IgM antibodies and viral culture.

12

Congenital Anomalies

Marium H. Smith and Janice L. Henderson

1. Which of the following represents the quadruple test result that would be considered a positive screening test for Down syndrome?

   A. Increased AFP, decreased unconjugated estriol, decreased hCG, increased inhibin A

   B. Decreased AFP, decreased unconjugated estriol, increased hCG, increased inhibin A

   C. Increased AFP, increased unconjugated estriol, decreased hCG, decreased inhibin A

   D. Decreased AFP, increased unconjugated estriol, increased hCG, increased inhibin A

   B Decreased AFP, decreased unconjugated estriol, increased hCG, increased inhibin A. See Table 12.1.

2. Which of the following is not true of omphalocele?

   A. Prognosis is dependent on the size of the lesion.

   B. Karyotyping is indicated.

   C. Damage to the small bowel most likely occurs as a result of chemical peritonitis.

   D. Omphalocele is frequently associated with other structural abnormalities.

   C Damage from chemical peritonitis may occur to the bowel in gastroschisis, not omphalocele. In omphalocele, the bowel is covered in membrane that protects it from the amniotic fluid, whereas in gastroschisis, the bowel is directly exposed to the fluid. Karyotyping is indicated in omphalocele because it may be associated with chromosomal

TABLE 12.1

Second Trimester Maternal Serum Test Results

Disorder	AFP	Estriol	hCG	Inhibin A
Neural tube defects	increased	—	—	—
Down syndrome	decreased	decreased	increased	increased
Trisomy 18	decreased	decreased	decreased	—

abnormalities, and a worse prognosis is associated with a larger lesion, especially if the liver is involved.

3. Which of the following gastrointestinal abnormalities is strongly associated with Down syndrome?

A. Duodenal atresia

B. Omphalocele

C. Esophageal atresia

D. Gastroschisis

> **A** Duodenal atresia, which is represented on ultrasound by the "double bubble sign," is strongly associated with Down syndrome.

4. Which of the following is a correct description of the nuchal translucency (NT)?

A. A second trimester ultrasound measurement, which is correctly performed at a cross-sectional view and clearly demonstrates the falx and the thalami

B. A common finding on prenatal ultrasound in infants affected with spina bifida

C. A measurement performed between 11½ and 13⅚ weeks that, when combined with maternal age and maternal serum hCG and PAPP–A, can be used to predict the likelihood of Down syndrome

D. A first-trimester measurement that is the most accurate way to perform ultrasonographic dating

> **C** Choice A refers to the view needed for biparietal diameter and head circumference when performing fetal biometry; choice B is Arnold-Chiari malformation; and choice D is incorrect since NT is not used for dating.

13

Endocrine Disorders of Pregnancy

Natalia Colón

1. An 18-year-old gravida 1 Para 0 at 9 weeks gestation presents to your clinic for a new OB visit. She has a history of type 1 diabetes mellitus (DM) since she was a teenager. Lab results show that her hemoglobin A1C is 10%. Her glucose checks reveal fasting levels in the 100s and 1-hour postprandial levels in the 200s. This patient's pregnancy is at risk for all of the following, *except:*

   A. IUGR
   B. Fetal death in utero
   C. Macrosomia
   D. Shoulder dystocia
   E. Oligohydramnios

   > **E** Fetuses of diabetic mothers are at risk for fetal structural malformations, especially in the cardiovascular system; spontaneous abortions, especially in poorly controlled diabetic patients; intrauterine growth restriction (IUGR) secondary to the presence of microvascular disease; and fetal demise in the third trimester. The diabetic pregnant patient is also at risk for polyhydramnios, macrosomia, and shoulder dystocia.

2. A 25-year-old gravida 3 Para 1011 at 31 weeks' gestation, with known gestational diabetes, presents to your office complaining of contractions every 3 to 5 minutes. You perform a vaginal exam and discover that the patient is 3 to 4 cm dilated. You decide to admit the patient and begin tocolysis as well as steroids

for fetal lung maturation. Which of the following medications is the tocolytic of choice in this patient?

A. Terbutaline

B. Indomethacin

C. Magnesium

D. Ritodrine

C When a patient with DM develops preterm labor, the choice of tocolytics is limited. Sympathomimetics (i.e., terbutaline sulfate, ritodrine hydrochloride) should be used with caution because they can exacerbate hyperglycemia and may cause ketoacidosis. Indomethacin may be used as long as maternal renal disease or poorly controlled hypertension is absent. Indomethacin should not be given after 32 weeks' gestation. Magnesium sulfate is the tocolytic agent of choice in the presence of preterm labor.

3. Fetuses of women with pregestational diabetes are at risk for all of the following congenital anomalies, *except*:

A. Hypoplastic left ventricle

B. Transposition of great vessels

C. Ventricular septal defect

D. Atrial septal defect

E. Pulmonary hypertension

E Congenital malformations are the most common contributor to perinatal mortality in pregnancies of women with pregestational DM. Some of these malformations include:

- Skeletal: The best example is sacral agenesis/caudal regression. It can be diagnosed up to 400 times more frequently in pregnancies complicated by diabetes.
- Cardiovascular anomalies are the most common congenital malformations in diabetic pregnancies, including transposition of the great vessels, ventricular and atrial septal defects, hypoplastic left ventricle, situs inversus, aortic anomalies, and complex anomalies. Fetal septal hypertrophy can also occur in the second half of the pregnancy.
- CNS anomalies. A 10-fold increase is seen in the incidence of CNS malformations in women with pregestational diabetes, including anencephaly,

holoprosencephaly, open spina bifida, microcephaly, encephalocele, and meningomyelocele.
- Malformations of the GI system are also found, including tracheoesophageal fistula, bowel atresia,
and imperforate anus.
- GU anomalies include absent kidneys (Potter's syndrome), polycystic kidneys, and double ureters.

4. A 35-year-old gravida 5 Para 2022 with gestational diabetes
mellitus has just delivered spontaneously at 39 weeks. Her
neonate is at risk for all of the following, *except:*

A. Hypocalcemia

B. Hypomagnesemia

C. Hypoglycemia

D. Hyperbilirubinemia

E. Anemia

E Twenty-five percent to 40% of infants of diabetic
mothers develop hypoglycemia during the first few hours
of life. The pathogenesis behind this involves stimulation
of the fetal pancreas in utero due to maternal hyperglycemia; this leads to fetal islet cell hypertrophy and beta
cell hyperplasia, which, in turn, leads to overproduction of
insulin by the fetus. Alterations in mineral metabolism are
common in infants of diabetic mothers, such as hypocalcemia and hypomagnesemia. One third of infants born to
diabetic mothers are polycythemic (hematocrit higher than
65%). Chronic intrauterine hypoxia leads to an increase in
erythropoietin production, with a resultant increase in red
blood cell production. Anemia is not a common complication for fetuses of diabetic mothers. Neonatal hyperbilirubinemia and neonatal jaundice occur more commonly in
the infants of diabetic mothers than in infants of nondia-
betic patients of comparable gestational age due to a delay
in in utero liver maturation among infants of diabetic
mothers with poor glycemic control.

5. Poorly controlled hyperthyroidism in pregnancy can result in
all of the following, *except:*

A. Pre-eclampsia

B. Congestive heart failure

C. Preterm labor

D. Preterm premature rupture of membranes

E. Intrauterine growth restriction

> **D** Thyrotoxicosis occurs in approximately 1 in 2,000 pregnancies. Poorly controlled hyperthyroidism can result in pre-eclampsia, thyroid storm, or congestive heart failure (CHF) for the mother, and preterm labor and delivery, IUGR, and stillbirth for the fetus.

6. A 25-year-old gravida 1 Para 0 at 36 weeks, with known hyperthyroidism, presents to your clinic with fever of 103°F, tachycardia, and agitation. Her blood pressure was noted to be 80/50. On lung exam, diffuse crackles are heard from the bases to the apices. The first line treatment for this patient is

A. Aggressive intravenous hydration

B. Intravenous beta blockers

C. PTU 450 mg every day

D. PTU 1,000 mg and potassium iodide

> **D** Thyroid storm is rarely seen during pregnancy. Heart failure, due to the long-term effects of T_4, is more likely encountered. Heart failure can be exacerbated by pregnancy-associated conditions, such as pre-eclampsia, anemia, or infection. In this state, the patient often has fever higher than 103°F, tachycardia, widened pulse pressure, and agitation. The patient may develop hypotension and cardiovascular collapse. Emergency states are treated with PTU 1 g and potassium iodide 1 g by mouth or nasogastric tube. With thyroid storm, IV beta blockers may be used, but these should be used cautiously with heart failure. Other supportive treatments include IV hydration and temperature control. Further assessment and treatment of other concomitant disorders are also crucial to reducing cardiac workload.

14

Hypertension in Pregnancy

Anya Bailis and Frank R. Witter

1. A 17-year-old gravida 1 para 0 at 38 2/7 weeks by dates and a first trimester sonogram presents to Labor and Delivery complaining of contractions. She denies any headaches, visual changes, abdominal pain or contractions, shortness of breath, or chest pain. Her past medical history is unremarkable. Her vital signs are as follows: temperature 37.0°C, pulse 88, respirations 16, blood pressure 150/84 and 155/90 on repeat, oxygen saturation of 99% on room air. On physical exam patient is well appearing, and periorbital edema is evident. Chest exam is unremarkable. No abdominal/fundal tenderness is palpated. Lower extremities have 1+ edema and 2+ deep tendon reflexes. Fetal membranes are intact, and her cervix is dilated 2 cm with 60% effacement, zero station. It is soft and anterior. The fetal heart rate tracing is reactive. Tocodynamometer shows rare contractions. CBC, complete metabolic profile, and coagulation parameters are within normal limits. Uric acid measures 7.4. Urine protein measures 2+ on urine dipstick. What is the best management plan?

A. Outpatient management with biweekly fetal testing until she goes into labor

B. Cesarean section

C. Induction of labor at 39 weeks

D. Immediate induction of labor

E. Hospital admission for observation with daily fetal testing

D This patient is term, with good dating and a favorable cervix (Bishop score of 9), and presents with criteria for mild pre-eclampsia. She would best be served by induction of labor. Unless she is showing signs of rapid progression to severe pre-eclampsia or DIC, or if the baby shows evidence of compromise, delivering emergently by cesarean section is unnecessary.

2. A 25-year-old presents to Labor and Delivery by ambulance after having had a witnessed seizure at home. On arrival the patient is obtunded and unable to answer questions. Her medical and prenatal histories are unknown. Her friend describes a sudden onset of generalized shaking, accompanied by loss of consciousness, lasting about 30 seconds before stopping abruptly. The friend thinks that the patient is about 7 months pregnant and doesn't recall any complaints before the seizure. Vital signs are as follows: temperature 36.8°C, pulse 80, respiratory rate 16, blood pressure 180/110. Fetal heart rate is in the 120s with minimal to moderate variability and no decelerations. Contractions are occasional. Physical exam is unremarkable, with the exception of a few bruises on the upper extremities. Cervical exam is 1 to 2 cm, 80% effacement, and zero station. Lab values are CBC, complete metabolic profile, and coagulation parameters are within normal limits. Uric acid is 7.9. Urine dip shows 4+ urine protein. An ultrasound shows a 31-week fetus with a biophysical profile of 8/10. What is the best course of management?

A. Magnesium, blood pressure control, and emergent cesarean section under general anesthesia

B. Magnesium, blood pressure control, and induction of labor

C. Magnesium, blood pressure control, and cesarean section with epidural anesthesia

D. Magnesium, blood pressure control, and observation

   B This patient presents with eclampsia. Protocol for eclampsia is seizure prophylaxis/treatment with magnesium, antihypertensives, and delivery. The patient's elevated blood pressures should be treated. Hydralazine and labetalol are first line medications. Because the patient is not currently seizing, and appears stable, and the fetal testing is reassuring, to attempt an induction of labor is safe. Her cervix is not overall favorable, however, and it is possible that the patient may, ultimately, require delivery by cesarean section.

3. A 32-year-old gravida 5 para 1-1-2-2 at 28 1/7 weeks' gestation presents to clinic for a routine prenatal visit. This patient has a past medical history of chronic hypertension that was first noted during her last pregnancy and did not resolve postpartum. During this pregnancy she has been taking Aldomet 250 mg bid, which has kept her pressures under control. Today her blood pressure reads at 152/86, with a recheck on her left side of 148/82. Her urine dip, which had been traced previously is 1+ today. She denies any symptoms and assures you that she has been taking her blood pressure medication. Her physical exam is unremarkable. Her CBC, complete metabolic profile, coagulation parameters, uric acid, and LDH are all within normal limits today. You send her to Labor and Delivery for monitoring and the tracing appears appropriate for gestational age. On ultrasound the baby is active and the amniotic fluid index is within normal limits. Which of the following is not an appropriate component of management?

A. 24-hour urine protein/calcium

B. Semiweekly fetal testing

C. Increasing Aldomet dosage

D. Weekly pre-eclampsia labs

E. Biweekly fetal growth ultrasounds

E Although she may be developing pre-eclampsia, this patient is only 28 weeks pregnant so she is managed differently than if she were term. Outpatient management with close monitoring is an acceptable way to follow her. Some would argue that a hospital admission for initial evaluation is a reasonable option as well. Weekly pre-eclampsia labs (CBC, CMP, uric acid), a 24-hour urine protein/calcium, and semiweekly fetal testing are all good methods of surveillance whether inpatient or outpatient. This patient is a chronic hypertensive in her third trimester, when blood pressures tend to elevate, so it is also reasonable to increase the dosage of her antihypertensive medication to bring down her BP as we try to buy some time for the baby to develop. Although an ultrasound for growth may be a good first step to assess fetal status, biweekly ultrasounds are unnecessary.

4. A 29-year-old gravida 2 para 2002 is postpartum day 1 status post a full-term spontaneous vaginal delivery. She had initially presented to Labor and Delivery from clinic where her blood pressures were noted to be elevated. She was diagnosed with pre-eclampsia based on persistently elevated blood pressures in the 150s/80s range and a 24-hour urine protein of 1 g. Her laboratory findings were always within normal limits. Because she was term and her cervix was favorable, it was decided to induce her labor. She was started on magnesium sulfate IV, and labor was induced quickly with Pitocin. The magnesium prophylaxis was continued postpartum. Approximately 8 hours after delivery, the patient's oxygen saturations were noted to be dropping although, subjectively, the patient was not dypneic. Fine crackles were auscultated bilaterally at the lung bases. Urine output is approximately 30 cc per hour. Which of the following is not appropriate at this time?

A. Turn off magnesium

B. Diuretics

C. Oxygen supplementation

D. Chest x-ray

E. Increasing IV fluids

E This patient has pulmonary edema until proven otherwise. Pre-eclampsia makes vessels leaky, causing fluid to escape from the intravascular space into the interstitial space. This extra fluid usually manifests as peripheral edema but may also generate pulmonary edema. In addition, the magnesium sulfate used for seizure prophylaxis can, in high levels, be responsible for pulmonary edema as well. This patient has low urine output due to intravascular depletion, but overall she is fluid overloaded and therefore should not be bolused with IV fluids. It will worsen her condition. A chest x-ray for evaluation, as well as supplemental oxygen, gentle diuresis, and discontinuation of the magnesium sulfate are all reasonable first steps. One might also consider central monitoring.

15

Cardiopulmonary Disorders of Pregnancy

Sasha Davidson and Ernest M. Graham

1. Of the following, which measurement of cardiac function decreases in pregnancy and reaches its nadir at the end of the second trimester?

   A. Cardiac output
   B. Heart rate
   C. Systemic blood pressure
   D. Maternal blood volume
   E. Preload

   C Blood volume increases 40% to 50% during normal pregnancy, due in part to estrogen-mediated activation of the renin-aldosterone axis. The rise in blood volume is greater than the increase in red blood cell mass, contributing to the fall in hemoglobin concentration. Cardiac output rises 30% to 50% above baseline by 20 to 24 weeks' gestation. It peaks by the end of the second trimester, after which it reaches a plateau until delivery. The change in cardiac output is mediated by increased preload due to the rise in blood volume, reduced afterload due to a fall in systemic vascular resistance, and a rise in the maternal heart rate by 10 to 15 beats per minute. Stroke volume increases during the first and second trimesters but declines in the third trimester due to caval compression by the gravid uterus.

2. Which of the following is *not* a predictor of maternal cardiac complications during pregnancy?

   A. Left ventricular function <40%
   B. Lone atrial fibrillation

C. New York Heart Association functional class I

D. Restrictive cardiomyopathy

E. Outflow tract obstruction

C See Table 15.1. The New York Heart Association functional class is often used as a predictor of outcome. Women with NYHA classes III and IV face a mortality rate upward of 7% and a morbidity rate of over 30%. These women should be strongly cautioned against pregnancy. In a study of 252 completed pregnancies in women with cardiac disease, five factors were found to be predictive of maternal cardiac complications. An updated risk index composed of the following four risk factors was shown to accurately predict a woman's chance of having adverse cardiac or neonatal complications: a previous cardiac event, cyanosis or poor functional class, left heart obstruction, and systemic ventricular dysfunction.

3. Of the following, which risk factor would *not* require prophylactic antibiotics to prevent bacterial endocarditis?

A. Prosthetic valve

B. Mitral valve prolapse with regurgitation

C. Acquired valve dysfunction

D. Pacemaker

E. Cyanotic congenital heart disease

TABLE 15.1

Predictors of Maternal Risk for Cardiac Complications

Previous cardiac events (heart failure, transient ischemic attack, stroke before pregnancy)
Previous arrhythmia requiring treatment
New York Heart Association functional class >2 or cyanosis
Valvular and outflow tract obstruction
Myocardial dysfunction (LVEF <40% or restrictive cardiomyopathy or hypertrophic cardiomyopathy)

From Siu SC, Sermer M, Harrison DA, et al. Risk and predictors for pregnancy-related complications in women with heart disease. *Circulation* 1997;96:2789–2794, with permission.

D High-risk categories include those patients with prosthetic cardiac valve, previous bacterial endocarditis, complex cyanotic congenital heart disease, and surgically constructed pulmonary shunts or conduits. Moderate risks include most other congenital cardiac malformations, acquired valve dysfunction, hypertrophic cardiomyopathy, mitral valve prolapse with valvular regurgitation, and/or thickened leaflets. No prophylaxis is needed in patients with isolated ostium secundum ASD, surgically repaired ASD, VSD, PDA; mitral valve prolapse without mitral regurgitation, thickened leaflets; innocent or physiologic murmurs; pacemakers or defibrillators; history of bypass surgery, Kawasaki's disease without valve dysfunction or history of rheumatic fever without valve dysfunction.

4. The presentation of peripartum cardiomyopathy is a gradual onset of symptoms of heart failure beginning during which of the following time periods?

   A. First 12 weeks
   B. 13 to 25 weeks
   C. 25 to 35 weeks
   D. After 36 weeks
   E. Before conception

   D Peripartum cardiomyopathy is a dilated cardiomyopathy of unknown cause that develops in late pregnancy or the first 6 months postpartum. The incidence is said to be approximately 1 in 1,300 to 1 in 15,000. Of the patients who survive, approximately 50% recover normal left heart function, but the others retain permanent cardiomyopathy. The mortality rate reported is 25% to 50%. Death from peripartum cardiomyopathy results from progressive CHF, thromboembolic events, and arrhythmias. Risk factors include multiparity, hypertension, cesarean section, increased maternal age, multiple gestations, and pre-eclampsia or eclampsia. Management of peripartum cardiomyopathy includes limiting activity, sodium restriction; medical therapy with afterload reducers, diuretics, inotropics, anticoagulants, or some combination of these; and, in cases of advanced disease, transplantation.

5. Which of the following has *not* been associated with the use of unfractionated heparin (UFH)?

A. Hemorrhage

B. Thrombocytopenia

C. Leukopenia

D. Maternal osteoporosis

E. HITT syndrome

> **C** UFH does not cross the placenta and is considered safer for the fetus. Its use, however, has been associated with maternal osteoporosis, hemorrhage, thrombocytopenia and/or thrombosis (HITT syndrome), and a high incidence of thromboembolic events with older generation mechanical valves. UFH may be administered IV or subcutaneously (SC) throughout pregnancy; when used SC, the recommended starting dose is 10,000 units twice daily. The appropriate dose adjustment of UFH is targeted to produce an activated partial thromboplastin time (aPTT) of 2.0 to 3.0 times the control level. High doses of UFH are often required to achieve the desired aPTT due to the hypercoagulable state associated with pregnancy. Parenteral infusions should be stopped at least 4 hours before cesarean sections. UFH can be reversed with protamine sulfate.

6. Which physiologic measurement of respiratory function is not altered during pregnancy?

A. Functional residual capacity (FRC)

B. Forced expiratory volume in 1 second (FEV$_1$)

C. Tidal volume

D. Minute ventilation

> **B** Elevation of the diaphragm due to increased abdominal girth causes a decrease in FRC, the resting position of the lungs at the end of a normal expiration. This decrease usually occurs during the second half of pregnancy. Despite the alteration in resting diaphragmatic position, diaphragm excursion is unaffected and so vital capacity is maintained. Airway function is normal during pregnancy, as FEV$_1$ (forced expiratory volume in the first second) and FEV$_1$/forced vital capacity (FVC) are normal. Resting

minute ventilation increases by 50%. Tidal volume increases by 30% to 40%, and forced expiratory volume and peak expiratory flow rate remain unchanged.

References
1. Siu SC, Sermer M, Harrison DA, et al. Risk and predictors for pregnancy-related complications in women with heart disease. *Circulation* 1997;96:2789–2794.

16

Renal, Hepatic, and Gastrointestinal Disorders and Systemic Lupus Erythematosus in Pregnancy

Thao Nguyen and Frank R. Witter

1. Chronic renal disease in pregnancy is associated with:

A. Perinatal mortality

B. Preterm birth

C. IUGR

D. All of the above

> **D** Chronic renal disease is associated with increased perinatal mortality, pre-eclampsia, eclampsia, preterm birth, and IUGR. Pregnant women with pre-existing renal disease are at risk for deterioration of renal function. Patients with moderate-to-severe renal insufficiency are at greatest risk for potentially irreversible deterioration of their renal function. Furthermore, chronic renal disease complicated by hypertension imposes a substantially increased risk to both patient and fetus.

2. Intrahepatic cholestasis of pregnancy:

A. Is rarely recurrent in subsequent pregnancies

B. Is less severely affected in subsequent pregnancies

C. Is not associated with fetal distress or fetal death

D. None of the above

D The recurrence rate of intrahepatic cholestasis is approximately 70%, with subsequent pregnancies more severely affected. One of the complications of intrahepatic cholestasis in pregnancy is intrauterine fetal demise. The risk increases progressively to term regardless of progression of symptoms. The cause of fetal demise is unknown and rarely happens before the last month of pregnancy.

3. Which of the following statements is false?

   A. Pregnancy does not alter the long-term prognosis of systemic lupus erythematosus (SLE) patients.

   B. Lupus flares during pregnancy are usually severe and involve cutaneous and articular symptoms.

   C. Transient lupus flares are more likely during pregnancy than at other times.

   D. SLE patients have increased risk of spontaneous abortion, IUGR, cesarean delivery, and fetal death.

   B Pregnancy does not appear to alter the long-term prognosis of most SLE patients. Transient lupus flares can occur during any trimester and are more likely to occur during pregnancy than at other times. These flares are usually mild and involve primarily cutaneous and articular symptoms. Patients with SLE have an increased risk of spontaneous abortion, premature birth, IUGR, fetal death, cesarean delivery, and pre-eclampsia. The risk of pre-eclampsia in SLE patients is further increased with history of antiphospholipid antibodies, renal disease, hypertension, or diabetes mellitus.

17

Hematologic Disorders of Pregnancy

K. Joseph Hurt

1. A 20-year-old Indonesian primigravida at 11 and 2/7 weeks' gestation presents for her initial obstetric visit. She has had no problems with the pregnancy and denies any medical conditions. Her registration labs show a hematocrit of 33%, MCV 77, and decreased hemoglobin A with elevated hemoglobin A2 and F on electrophoresis. You plan to offer her all of the following management options, *except*:

   A. 1 mg folate supplementation per day
   B. Paternal DNA testing
   C. Chorionic villus sampling/fetal DNA testing
   D. 120 mg per day of elemental iron supplementation
   E. Frequent ultrasounds and nonstress testing

   D This laboratory data in an Asian woman strongly suggest beta thalassemia. Although the mother is asymptomatic, she is in fact anemic. Folic acid can increase term hemoglobin concentrations, though iron supplementation is unnecessary in the absence of a coexisting iron-deficiency anemia. She should have close follow-up with regular ultrasounds to assess fetal growth and antenatal testing in the third trimester to evaluate fetal well-being. The race of the father and the results of paternal testing for hemoglobinopathies should be assessed. Based on the results of paternal screening, the couple may decide to pursue fetal DNA testing. Genetic counseling would be helpful in educating the parents and helping them develop reasonable expectations for this pregnancy as well as identifying their genetic risk for future children.

2. A 19-year-old primigravida at 36 to 2/7 weeks' gestation presents to Labor and Delivery with nausea and vomiting for the past 24 hours. She has a headache and has been unable to tolerate any food for 1 day but believes that her symptoms are due to the same viral illness that has made her colleagues sick at work over the past week. You send HELLP labs that are all within normal limits, except the platelets that are 98,000/μL. In addition to an NST, which of these is the best intervention?

A. Growth ultrasound to evaluate for growth restriction

B. Antepartum admission for observation and serial laboratory work

C. Treat with antiemetics and intravenous fluids then discharge home

D. Begin dexamethasone treatments to improve platelet counts

E. Start an immediate induction of labor

C Thrombocytopenia is defined as platelets less than 150,000/μL. Gestational thrombocytopenia affects 5% of all pregnancies and is the most frequent cause of all pregnancy-associated platelets decreases. Thrombocytopenia is a benign diagnosis of exclusion and need not be treated. To make the diagnosis, the following criteria should be met: (a) The patient had a normal prepregnancy platelet count; (b) the platelet count is at least 70,000 or greater; (c) no previous history exists of thrombocytopenia except during pregnancies; and (d) no bleeding, bruising, or similar symptoms are present. No intervention is necessary except to regularly monitor platelet count and check for normal postpartum neonatal and maternal platelets (most rise to normal levels by 6 weeks after delivery). The primary intervention, in this case, should be a thorough history and physical exam, with antiemetics and IV hydration to prevent or correct dehydration. The symptoms of headache, nausea, and vomiting are concerning in a nearly term patient, but they may be nonspecific symptoms of many conditions. The patient should be discharged home with strict labor and pre-eclamptic warnings with consideration given to obtaining a 24-hour urine protein. NST should be recorded for all third-trimester patients on labor and delivery and a BPP performed if the result is not reactive. Corticosteroid treatments are occasionally used to boost extremely low platelet counts in HELLP patients but not for gestational thrombocytopenia. An induction of labor, especially in a preterm gestation, would not be indicated.

3. A 34-year-old gravida 3, para 1142, with a history of deep vein thrombosis while taking oral contraceptive pills, is referred from her primary care doctor at 9 weeks' gestational age. She has had one first trimester elective abortion and three spontaneous miscarriages in the early second trimester. She has never had a thrombophilia workup. Which of the following needs to be included on your differential diagnosis?

A. Factor V Leiden mutation

B. Protein C or protein S deficiency

C. Lupus anticoagulant or anticardiolipin antibody

D. Hyperhomocysteinemia or MTHFR deficiency

E. All of the above

E Normal pregnancy is a hypercoagulable state, with a fivefold increased risk for DVT and PE. Even more concerning is the exacerbation of undiagnosed/underlying thrombophilias that pregnancy may cause. Routine screening is not recommended, but a patient with history of DVT or second-trimester losses should be thoroughly evaluated. All of the listed conditions or mutations are associated with increased maternal thrombosis. More than half of DVTs are detected before 15 weeks' gestation, and patients with increased risk should be examined carefully because most go undiagnosed. Other inherited thrombophilias include prothrombin gene (G20210A) mutation, 4G/4G PAI-1 mutation, or antithrombin deficiency. Acquired risk factors include increasing age, obesity, high parity, cesarean section, bed rest or immobility, trauma, pre-eclampsia, and smoking.

4. For the patient in question 3, which of the following is the best treatment recommendation?

A. Immediate 1 mg/kg of enoxaparin every 12 hours

B. Immediate 40 mg enoxaparin per day

C. Immediate 1,000 units heparin every 12 hours

E. Wait for the results before initiating therapy

E Women with previous idiopathic or pregnancy/OCP-related venous thromboembolism deserve immediate antepartum and postpartum (6 weeks) prophylaxis. Choice A is the therapeutic, rather than prophylactic, dose of LMWH. Choice B is prophylactic, but twice daily dosing is preferred in pregnancy due to the increased creatinine clearance. Choice C is the second-trimester dosing for UFH. Waiting till the second trimester, as in choice D, neglects early DVT risk. For UFH dosing, monitor the aPTT/aPTTr. For LMWH, monitor the antifactor Xa levels. The anticoagulant may be started after the blood for the patient's thrombophilia workup has been sent for testing. If her testing confirms a high-risk thrombophilia, such as antithrombin deficiency, Factor V Leiden, or prothrombin mutation, she could then be started on therapeutic anticoagulation. Two or more episodes of VTE and women on chronic anticoagulation for mechanical heart valves or atrial fibrillation should also receive the higher therapeutic dosing. Neither unfractionated nor low molecular weight heparin cross the placenta and are safe for the developing fetus in all trimesters. Only at the time of induction or cesarean section should anticoagulation be stopped; it may be wise to transition to unfractionated heparin from enoxaparin near term.

5. A 24-year-old African American gravida 2, para 1001 at 23 to 3/7 weeks' gestation comes to her regular clinic visit. She denies any obstetric complaints but does report increasing fatigue, reduced exercise tolerance (feeling winded after one flight of stairs), and recent cravings for ice chips. Her registration labs at 9 weeks showed a hematocrit of 37, MCV of 83, and hemoglobin electrophoresis type AA2. She has no personal or family history of hematologic disorders, has never experienced similar problems in previous pregnancies, and has been taking chewable over-the-counter multivitamins since she became pregnant. Which of the following pieces of information would be least useful in formulating an appropriate treatment plan?

A. Hematocrit/hemoglobin level

B. Mean corpuscular volume

C. Prepregnancy ferritin level

D. Total iron-binding capacity

E. Current ferritin level

D Maternal blood volumes may increase as much as 20% to 100% in pregnancy. Plasma volume peaks around 30 to 34 weeks, whereas RBC mass increases progressively until term. The resulting mismatch in plasma volume and RBC mass can produce the physiologic anemia of pregnancy. Determining whether this patient has normal hematologic changes versus symptomatic anemia (with pica) warrants further investigation. A CBC would give the hemoglobin level (to assess the degree of anemia) along with an MCV to indicate the need for further iron studies. Ferritin levels closely parallel body iron stores and are the best indicator of maternal iron deficiency. If the ferritin level is less than 12 mg/mL, the diagnosis of iron-deficiency anemia is made. If the iron stores are normal, consider thalassemia. Because this woman appears to have entered pregnancy with borderline anemia, she may require 60 to 120 mg elemental iron rather than the recommended 30 mg iron supplementation per day. In this case, 325 mg of ferrous sulfate, ferrous gluconate, or ferrous fumarate supplements may be indicated two or three times a day along with a stool softener to prevent severe constipation. The serum iron level and TIBC may be lowered in normal pregnancies in the absence of anemia, though they are typical components of a full iron-deficiency anemia workup.

18

Red Blood Cell Alloimmunization

Janyne E. Althaus

1. In which of the following situations should RhoGAM be given?

A. Rh− woman, −D antibodies, with Rh− husband by serology, at 28 weeks

B. Rh− woman, +D antibodies, after amniocentesis

C. Rh− woman with +Lewis antibodies at 28 weeks

D. Rh+ woman, −D antibodies after amniocentesis

E. Rh− woman, −D antibodies who just delivered an Rh− neonate.

C Only Rh− women need RhoGAM, so choice D is incorrect. Rh− women who are not exposed to the D antigen are not at risk, so scenarios A and E do not require RhoGAM. As RhoGAM is preventative only, the woman in scenario B will not benefit from RhoGAM because she has already been sensitized. Although the woman in scenario C already has a red cell antibody, she is still at risk for alloimmunization to the D antigen and should therefore receive RhoGAM.

2. Which of the following red cell antigens does not lead to hydrops fetalis?

A. Lea

B. D

C. Kell

D. Duffy

E. c

A A good sentence to remember is "Duffy dies, Kell kills but Lewis lives." All Rh antigens (c,C,D,e,E) can lead to hydrops.

3. At her first prenatal visit at 8 weeks, an Rh− woman with a history of a previous miscarriage is found to have a +D antibody titer of 1:16. The next step is to:

   A. Repeat maternal antibody screen in 4 to 6 weeks.
   B. Perform amniocentesis at 15 to 18 weeks.
   C. Determine paternal red cell phenotype.
   D. Sonogram to confirm gestational age
   E. Administer RhoGAM.

   D Initial sonogram to confirm gestational age is essential to properly manage an Rh sensitized patient. Once the critical titer of 1:16 has been reached, an Rh+ fetus will be at risk and titers will no longer be useful. Paternal cell phenotype will need to be established following the sonogram. Amniocentesis is not performed until paternal phenotype is determined or if it is unknown. RhoGAM is of no benefit in an Rh sensitized patient.

19

Surgical Disease and Trauma in Pregnancy

Mary Ellen Pavone and Nancy A. Hueppchen

1. Which of the following statements is true?

A. Because recent abdominal surgery has been associated with an increased chance of an incisional dehiscence, all patients who have recently had abdominal surgery should be delivered via cesarean section.

B. Teratogenic risks of radiation are highest between 8 and 15 weeks of gestation.

C. Optimal timing for surgery is during the first trimester because later timing has been associated with preterm labor.

D. All pregnant women who undergo surgery should also receive tocolytic agents to prevent preterm labor.

> **B** Recent abdominal surgery is not a contraindication for undergoing a vaginal delivery. Optimal timing for surgery is during the second trimester. Surgery during the first trimester carries an increased risk of spontaneous abortion because of disruption of the corpus luteum. Preterm labor and poor operative exposure make surgery difficult during the third trimester. Current data do not support the routine use of tocolytic agents in women who undergo surgery.

2. A 23-year-old gravida 1 P0 at 16 weeks' gestation presents to Labor and Delivery with acute right lower quadrant pain, nausea, and vomiting. On exam, she is not contracting. The fetal heart rate is appropriate for gestational age. Her cervical exam shows a closed, noneffaced cervix. What additional tests should be ordered to help establish a diagnosis?

A. No other tests should be ordered. The patient should be consented for immediate surgery.

B. Pelvic ultrasound

C. General surgery consult

D. CT scan

> **B** A pelvic ultrasound may be helpful in diagnosing a ruptured corpus luteum or ovarian torsion and should be ordered if the patient is otherwise stable. It should be ordered before undergoing a CT scan or calling a general surgery consult.

3. You, the chief resident on Labor and Delivery, receive a call from the emergency department that a woman about 36 weeks' gestation has been found in cardiac arrest and is being transported to your hospital. All of the following statements are true, *except:*

   A. The uterus should be deflected to the left during chest compressions to alleviate compression of abdominal and pelvic vessels.

   B. An emergency cesarean delivery should be performed only if a viable fetus is found.

   C. Common causes of maternal cardiac arrest include pulmonary embolism, amniotic fluid embolism, and stroke.

   D. Vasopressors should be avoided, if possible, because they cause a decrease in uteroplacental perfusion.

   > **B** Because a pregnant uterus may impede maternal resuscitative efforts, a cesarean delivery may be performed even if a nonviable fetus is suspected.

4. You are called to assess a 33-year-old Para 1-0-0-1 at 35 0/7 weeks' gestation on the burn unit who has sustained a 30% total body surface area burn after a house fire. You recommend:

   A. A daily nonstress test to assess fetal well-being; continue routine treatment for the mother

   B. A daily biophysical profile to assess fetal well-being; continue routine treatment for the mother

   C. Urgent delivery

   D. A complete fetal ultrasound; if no abnormalities are found, routine fetal surveillance and routine maternal treatment

C Urgent delivery in all term or near-term pregnant patients with extensive thermal injuries is the treatment of choice because of a high rate of maternal and fetal mortality. Because of the extent of the maternal injury, continuing to monitor the pregnancy is unsafe, even using fetal surveillance, including the nonstress test, biophysical profile, or complete fetal ultrasound.

5. Physiologic changes in pregnancy include all of the following, *except:*

   A. A relative leukocytosis
   B. Decreased hematocrit
   C. Hyperalbuminemia
   D. Increased plasma volume

   C Hypoalbuminemia, not hyperalbuminemia, occurs and predisposes pregnant women to edema.

20

Postpartum Care and Breast-Feeding

Mary Ellen Pavone, Scott C. Purinton, and Scott M. Petersen

1. All of the following are true regarding the management of postpartum hemorrhage, *except:*

   A. Causes include uterine atony, vaginal, cervical, or perineal laceration, and retained products of conception.

   B. Methylergonovine maleate is contraindicated in patients with asthma.

   C. Risk factors for developing postpartum hemorrhage include multiple gestation, grand multiparity, prolonged labor, oxytocin augmentation, and advanced maternal age.

   D. Vaginal bleeding after a vaginal delivery is prevented by uterine contraction.

   B Methylergonovine maleate is contraindicated in patients with elevated blood pressures, including patients with pre-eclampsia and hypertension.

2. A 19-year-old G1P1001 had an uncomplicated spontaneous vaginal delivery. She presents to Labor and Delivery triage with a temperature of 39.0°C on postpartum day 9 and fundal tenderness. She is diagnosed with postpartum endomyometritis. Which of the following organisms would most likely be the cause of her infection?

   A. *Group B Streptococcus*

   B. *Escherichia coli*

   C. *Klebsiella pneumoniae*

   D. *Chlamydia trachomatis*

D The primary pathogen involved in endomyometritis differs depending on the postpartum day that the infection occurs. In general, postpartum days 1 to 2: group A Streptococcus; postpartum days 3 to 4: enteric organisms; and postpartum day 7 or greater: *C. trachomatis.*

3. Which of the following is true regarding immunizations during the postpartum period?

A. All vaccines should be given before a mother begins breast-feeding.

B. All rubella nonimmune mothers should be given a monovalent rubella vaccine before discharge because it is more cost-effective than giving the MMR vaccine.

C. Giving hepatitis B vaccines during the postpartum period is contraindicated.

D. Women who are Rh− should receive Rh immunoglobulin within 72 hours of delivery of an Rh+ infant.

D Women who are Rh− should receive Rh immunoglobulin within 72 hours of delivery of an Rh+ infant to avoid Rh sensitization. The use of monovalent rubella vaccine is no longer considered appropriate because MMR is more cost-effective and because many of the women without immunity to rubella also lack immunity to rubeola. Breast-feeding is not a contraindication to administering vaccinations. Giving the hepatitis B vaccine is not contraindicated during the postpartum period.

4. All of the following are strict contraindications to breast-feeding, *except:*

A. Chronic hepatitis B

B. Active herpetic lesions on the breast

C. Active maternal cocaine use

D. Maternal use of lithium

A Chronic hepatitis B is not a strict contraindication to breast-feeding if the infant has received hepatitis B immunoglobulin and the hepatitis B vaccine. However, women who have had acute hepatitis B infection during pregnancy should not breast-feed.

5. Which of the following statements regarding contraception in breast-feeding mothers is true?

A. Progestin-based contraception can affect the quality of breast milk and therefore should be avoided in breast-feeding mothers.

B. Lactational amenorrhea is up to 95% to 99% effective if strict criteria are followed.

C. Combined estrogen-progestin contraceptives do not affect the quality and quantity of breast milk and therefore can be started in the immediate postpartum period.

D. The mean time to ovulation in mothers who breast-feed is 45 days.

B Lactational amenorrhea has been shown to provide 95% to 99% protection in the first 6 months postpartum if the following strict criteria are followed: Feedings need to be every 4 hours during the day and every 6 hours at night, and supplemental feedings should not exceed 5% to 10% of the total.

21

Obstetric Anesthesia

Jennifer E. Cho and Donald H. Penning

1. A 26-year-old gravida 1 Para 0 who is currently 39 weeks pregnant comes in with spontaneous rupture of membranes with thick meconium and is 2 cm dilated, 80% effaced, and at zero station. Pitocin augmentation is started. During the course of her labor, variable decelerations occur down to the 100s and return to baseline with position changes down to the 100s. She receives an epidural and has no further decelerations until several hours later, when she is 8 cm dilated. A fetal heart rate deceleration occurs with a contraction down to the 60s for 4 minutes, unresponsive to position changes, pitocin cessation, and terbulaline. In the rush to roll the patient back to the operating room for a stat cesarean section, her epidural tip falls to the floor. What is the most appropriate form of anesthesia for this case?

   A. Epidural
   B. Spinal
   C. General
   D. Pudendal nerve block

   C Management of fetal heart decelerations include positioning the patient on her side to displace weight off the aorta and increase venous return, as well as providing oxygen to increase her oxygen reserve. Deep knee chest positioning may also provide resolution of the decelerations. Pitocin is turned off and terbutaline may be administered because uterine contractions are ischemic, and hyperstimulation or uterine tetany may lead to decreased placental perfusion. If the fetal heart rate does not return to its baseline after several minutes, a stat cesarean section is indicated.

In stat cesarean sections, if the patient does not have an epidural, general anesthesia is administered due to the emergent nature of the procedure. Ideally, an epidural is preferred because it allows the patient to be awake while her baby is born as well as provide adequate relief during and after the operation. However, an epidural requires more time to place the catheter, whereas general anesthesia can be quickly administered. Although general anesthesia carries with it an increased likelihood of aspiration and the disadvantage of being unconscious at the moment of birth, in an emergent situation, the decreased time with general makes it the preferred method of anesthesia.

In this scenario, although the patient has an epidural, it has been contaminated. Using it will lead to increased risk of infection and meningitis, and placing another epidural will take too much time. Therefore, general anesthesia is the most appropriate form of anesthesia indicated in this case.

2. Three patients are admitted to Labor and Delivery at approximately the same time. The first one is an HIV-positive woman who is gravida 5 Para 4004 and is 38 weeks pregnant, with a viral load of 100 and CD4 count of 314. She is 4 cm dilated and rates her pain as 10 out of 10. The second patient is a Hispanic woman, gravida 1 Para 0 at 39 4/7 weeks, who has confirmed rupture of membranes and is 1 cm dilated. She is yelling for pain medications with her contractions, which are coming every 5 minutes. Last, a 21-year-old with a severe case of antiphospholipid syndrome on anticoagulation therapy comes in 8 cm dilated with a bulging bag on examination, and in extreme discomfort. All three women are requesting an epidural, and only one anesthesiologist is on call. How would you prioritize the order in which these women receive an epidural, if they are to get one at all?

A. First HIV patient, second Hispanic patient, third antiphospholipid syndrome patient

B. Hispanic patient only. The HIV and antiphospholipid patients should not get an epidural.

C. First antiphospholipid patient, second HIV patient, third Hispanic patient

D. First Hispanic patient, second antiphospholipid patient. The HIV patient should not get an epidural.

E. First HIV patient, second Hispanic patient. The antiphospholipid patient should not get an epidural.

E Several contraindications preclude an epidural placement, among them being patient refusal, coagulopathies, refractory hypotension, increased intracranial pressure, back infections, and extensive surgeries of the back. Patients who take anticoagulation therapy, or those who are prone to bleeding, are not eligible for an epidural because an increased risk of a hematoma is present. Those who have refractory hypotension may have problems with an epidural placement, because receiving medication through an epidural may commonly cause an episode of hypotension and decreased placental perfusion. Women with increased intracranial pressures may have herniation of cerebral contents with an epidural. Finally, an increased risk of meningitis is present with epidurals in parturients having pre-existing back infections or bacteremia.

Keeping these contraindications in mind, the only patient who should not receive an epidural is the patient with antiphospholipid syndrome receiving anticoagulation therapy. The parturient with antiphospholipid syndrome may not receive an epidural because she has an increased risk of forming a hematoma from the procedure. However, she can receive pain relief using other methods, such as repeated doses of intravenous pain medications, such as Toradol or Stadol. Nerve blocks, such as a paracervical or pudendal block, can also be administered as the patient progresses in her labor and delivery as well. Although an epidural is the preferred method of pain control in the United States, other effective means are available for providing adequate relief to the parturient.

Of the two remaining patients, no reason should prevent anyone with well-controlled HIV to receive an epidural, unless they are floridly bacteremic, have low platelets, and are predisposed to bleeding, or have some other contraindication. Because the patient is gravida 5, extremely uncomfortable, and more likely to progress quickly to delivery than the Hispanic patient, the HIV patient should first get the epidural.

The Hispanic patient should be next in line for an epidural, because she is only 1 cm dilated and this is her first child; she will not be delivering soon. While waiting, one can consider giving her intravenous fentanyl or morphine or another agent to temporarily provide pain relief.

3. A 34-year-old woman who is 41 weeks pregnant has come in for an induction of labor with a favorable cervix. She declines any anesthesia. She progresses and becomes fully dilated. After 2 hours, she has made good progression and fetal station at +3. The fetal heart-tracing shows severe variable decelerations, and forceps are applied to expedite delivery. The patient agrees to a pudendal nerve block at this time due to the physician's insistence. What is the most concerning and common complication from placing a pudendal nerve block using lidocaine at this point in the delivery process?

A. Injecting anesthesia into the baby's scalp

B. Further fetal bradycardia

C. Lidocaine toxicity in the mother

D. Inadequacy of the pudendal block

C Lidocaine toxicity in the mother. In a forceps-assisted delivery, one needs to block the nerves that carry the pain pathways from the second stage of labor, namely the sacral nerves. A pudendal block is most likely to be used, because it blocks the pudendal nerve (S2 to S4). A paracervical block would not be helpful in a patient who is fully dilated, because there would be no more cervix left to inject the anesthetic. Local injection is mainly used for repairs of lacerations or episiotomies and will likely not be used in a forceps-assisted delivery.

With a pudendal block, minimal risk exists of injecting the anesthesia into the baby's scalp with a pudendal block, because the needle is angled away from the head on application, aimed posteriorly toward the ischial spines. There may be rapid absorption of the anesthetic agent, in this case lidocaine, which may lead to several maternal complications. The most common side effects are neurologic, such as tremor, light-headedness, drowsiness, and, in rare cases, seizures. One may have cardiovascular and gastrointestinal effects as well, such as sinus slowing, hypotension, nausea, vomiting, and even asystole and shock. Fetal bradycardia is not commonly seen with a pudendal block. A pudendal block may be ineffective in about half the cases that it is applied.

In this scenario, the patient desires to tolerate the pains of labor without any anesthesia and agrees to a pudendal block only toward the end. Thus, scenario D is not a major concern. Injecting into the baby's scalp or giving further fetal bradycardia is not likely. However, the mother may have side effects from the lidocaine, if it is rapidly absorbed.

4. A 27-year-old woman, para 1001, just delivered a healthy baby boy. The delivery was uncomplicated, and the woman had no lacerations that needed to be repaired. Her labor pain was adequately controlled with an epidural, which was pulled out after the delivery. She had an uncomplicated postpartum course and left the hospital in stable condition on the day after her delivery. The next day, she presents to the Labor and Delivery suite with complaints of a pounding frontal headache, which has not been responsive to adequate bed rest, hydration, Tylenol, or Motrin. She states that the headache is better when she lies down and worse when she sits or stands. What is the appropriate order in which this headache can be managed?

A. More Motrin and Tylenol

B. CT and MRI of the head

C. Caffeine, blood patch

D. Intravenous fluids

C Caffeine, blood patch. Several side effects exist from an epidural, the most common of which is the spinal headache. This occurs in the majority of cases in which the dural membranes are punctured during the placement of an epidural. Some hypothesize that the headache occurs due to continued leak of CSF leading to decreased intracranial pressure and causing the brain to have traction along the skull, activating the pain-sensitive meninges. Alternatively, the headache is thought to be caused by reflex vasodilation due to decreased intracranial pressure. Common symptoms of a spinal headache include exacerbation of the headache with position changes and a throbbing headache in the frontal or occipital region. In this scenario, a likely explanation for this patient's headache is dural puncture during her epidural catheter placement.

Initial management includes hydration, bed rest, and oral analgesics. If this is not adequate, then caffeine products or IV caffeine can be administered. An effective means of controlling the headache is the blood patch, which involves the injection of 15 to 25 mL of autologous blood into the epidural space near the initial puncture site. This blood then forms a clot around the leak, thus sealing it off and relieving the headache. Although the blood patch is highly effective, it is often not the first-line management for a headache and is done when other options have not worked. If caffeine and a blood patch do not prove to be effective, other diagnoses should be investigated. Depending on the situation, a CT and MRI of the head could be done to see if any neurologic abnormalities are present.

In the presented scenario, the patient has already tried the initial management of oral hydration, bed rest, and analgesics without any relief. The next step would be to encourage caffeine intake and a blood patch. The MRI and CT are not indicated as the next step in the management of this woman's headache, and oral analgesics and hydration have been proved to be ineffective in the patient thus far.

22

Anatomy of the Female Pelvis

Kimberly B. Fortner

1. Below the arcuate line, the abdominal wall is thought of in layers. Moving from outside to inside, the layers are as follows: skin, Camper's and Scarpa's fascias, and then:

A. Internal oblique, external oblique, transverse abdominus, transversalis fascia, peritoneum

B. Internal oblique, transverse abdominus, external oblique, transversalis fascia, peritoneum

C. External oblique, internal oblique, transverse abdominus, transversalis fascia, peritoneum

D. External oblique, transverse abdominus, external oblique, transversalis fascia, peritoneum

C The aponeuroses of the external oblique, internal oblique, and transverse abdominus muscles comprise the rectus sheath. The anterior rectus sheath is anatomically different above and below the **arcuate line.** The arcuate line (linea semicircularis, semilunar fold of Douglas) is located midway between the umbilicus and symphysis pubis. **Below the arcuate line,** the layers of the abdominal wall are as follows: skin, Camper's and Scarpa's fascias, then aponeuroses of the external obliques, internal obliques, transverse abdominus, followed by the transversalis fascia and peritoneum. **Above the arcuate line,** the anterior rectus sheath is composed of the aponeuroses of the external oblique and ventral half of the internal oblique muscles. The posterior rectus sheath is composed of the aponeuroses of the dorsal half of the internal oblique and transverse abdominus muscles.

2. The pelvic diaphragm is a coordinated muscle group called the *levator ani*. The muscles included as part of this structure are as follows:

A. Ischiococcygeus, pubococcygeus, and iliococcygeus

B. Puborectalis, pubococcygeus, and iliococcygeus

C. Puborectalis, ischiococcygeus, and pubococcygeus

D. Ischiocavernosus, bulbocavernosus, and ischiococcygeus

> **B** The **muscles of the pelvic diaphragm** comprise the levator ani and coccygeal muscles. These are covered by the superior and inferior fascias (Fig. 22.1). **Levator ani muscles** include the **puborectalis** that arises from the inner surface of the pubic bones and inserts into the rectum. Some fibers form a sling around the posterior aspect of the rectum. The **pubococcygeus** arises from the pubic bones and inserts into the anococcygeal raphe and superior aspect of the coccyx. The **iliococcygeus** arises from the **arcus tendineus levator ani** and inserts into the anococcygeal raphe and coccyx. The **coccygeus muscle** arises from the ischial spine and inserts into the coccyx and lowest area of the sacrum. It lies cephalad to the sacrospinous ligament.

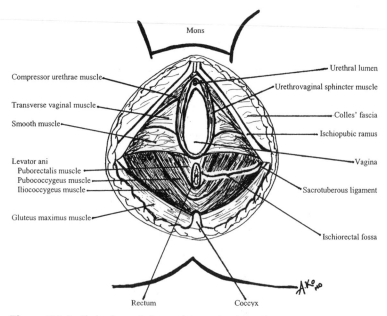

Figure 22.1. Skeletal muscle layer of the perineal membrane.

3. In regard to lymphatic drainage of the pelvic structures, all of the following pairings are correct, *except:*

   A. Vulva and vagina drain to the inguinofemoral lymph nodes.

   B. Vulva and vagina drain to pelvic (hypogastric, obturator, and external iliac) and para-aortic lymph nodes.

   C. Cervix drains to pelvic nodes (hypogastric, obturator, and external iliac).

   D. Cervix drains to common iliac and para-aortic lymph nodes.

   E. Uterus drains to pelvic (hypogastric, obturator, and external iliac) and para-aortic lymph nodes.

   B The lymphatic drainage of the pelvis typically follows the vessels and nerves. The vulva and lower vagina drain to the inguinofemoral lymph nodes and then on to the external iliac nodes. The cervix drains through the cardinal ligaments to the pelvic nodes (hypogastric, obturator, and external iliac), and then to the common iliac and para-aortic lymph nodes. The uterus drains through the broad ligament and intraperitoneal ligament to the pelvic and para-aortic lymph nodes. The ovaries drain to the pelvic and para-aortic lymph nodes.

23

Perioperative Care and Complications of Gynecologic Surgery

M. Shoma Datta and Robert E. Gutman

1. You schedule a new patient for a total abdominal hysterectomy due to symptomatic fibroids. Her uterus is approximately 24 weeks in size. She is a 43-year-old African American with a history of two previous abdominal myomectomy procedures. She has a 5-year history of well-controlled hypertension, is currently taking hydrochlorothiazide, and is otherwise healthy. She tells you that her "throat swells up" when she takes penicillin. The patient gives you a history of heavy cigarette smoking for 10 years, but she quit 7 years ago. Which of the following statements is *false?*

   A. She should be given metronidazole 1 g IV before surgery for antibiotic prophylaxis.

   B. Postsurgery, she should receive metronidazole every 8 hours to complete a 24-hour course to help prevent postoperative infections.

   C. A perioperative beta blocker should be added to her regimen for cardiovascular protection.

   D. She is at increased risk for ureteral, bowel, and bladder injuries secondary to the size of her uterus and previous surgeries.

   B Recent updated guidelines by the American College of Obstetricians and Gynecologists (ACOG) indicate that metronidazole 1 g IV or tinidazole 2 g PO (4 to 12 hours before surgery) are the antibiotics of choice in women with a history of immediate hypersensitivity to penicillin. Antibiotics should be administered within an hour before the incision. If a procedure is particularly long, additional intraoperative doses of an antibiotic may be needed, given at intervals of one or two times the half-life of the drug, to maintain adequate levels throughout the operation. An additional dose may be appropriate in cases with an increased blood loss (greater than 1,500 mL). Postsurgery doses of antibiotics have not been shown to prevent infection. Choice C is correct because perioperative beta blockade appears to decrease the incidence of myocardial events and overall long-term cardiac mortality after major surgery in patients at intermediate or high risk. Beta-1 blocking agents are typically recommended, starting days or weeks before elective surgery, with doses tapered postoperatively. Choice D is also correct. Risk factors for surgical injuries include malignant tumors, endometriosis, bulky uteri, and previous abdominal surgery.

2. During a complicated abdominal hysterectomy, you have difficulty isolating the left infundibulopelvic ligament due to extensive adhesive disease. You are able to place a clamp around the pedicle at the level of the pelvic brim when you realize you have unintentionally injured the ureter at your pedicle. On close inspection, the trauma has caused a partial transection of the ureter without crush or thermal damage. The next best step in management is:

A. Expectant management

B. Place a ureteral stent and manage expectantly with a Foley catheter in place.

C. Complete the transection and perform a transureter-oureterostomy.

D. Repair the defect with absorbable suture and place a ureteral stent.

E. Complete the transection and perform a ureteroneocystostomy.

D An injury to the ureter at the level of the pelvic brim is one of the most common sites of injury, usually during division of the infundibulopelvic ligament for hysterectomy. The next appropriate step is a repair of the defect or an end-to-end repair or ureteroureterostomy of this ureter. The defect must be repaired, and at this high level in the pelvis, a ureteroneocystostomy would be difficult, thus ruling out the remaining answer options.

3. A 41-year-old woman has undergone a total abdominal hysterectomy and bilateral salpingo-oophorectomy for treatment of symptomatic uterine leiomyomata. She was discharged home on postoperative day 3 without complication. She returns to the emergency department on postoperative day 12 with refractory nausea and bilious vomiting. Her heart rate is 82 beats per minute; regular, respiratory rate 21 per minute; and blood pressure 130/65 mm Hg. She is afebrile, her abdomen is moderately distended and diffusely tender, and intermittent high-pitched bowel sounds are present. The incision is clean, dry, and intact. Laboratory values show a hemoglobin of 11 mg/dL, white blood cell count of 13,600/mm^3, and platelet count of 305,000/mm^3. Serum electrolytes, BUN, and creatinine are normal. A left lateral decubitus film of her abdomen shows air-fluid levels. An upright film shows scant gas in the distal rectum and none under the diaphragm. What is the most likely diagnosis?

A. Intraoperative bowel injury

B. Diverticulosis

C. Inflammatory bowel disease

D. Small bowel obstruction

E. Incarcerated hernia

D Small bowel obstruction. See explanation for question 4.

4. What is the most appropriate management for the patient previously discussed?

A. Expectant management

B. Nasogastric tube decompression

C. Abdominal CT with contrast

D. Immediate re-exploration

E. Enema

F. Rectal suppository

B Nasogastric tube decompression. Small bowel obstruction is an infrequent postoperative complication of benign gynecologic surgery. Postoperative small bowel obstruction is due to a physical barrier, whereas an ileus results from neurogenic failure of peristalsis. Patients will usually present with vomiting, abdominal discomfort, and distention. Bowel sounds may be absent or hypoactive and high-pitched, but the condition is difficult to distinguish in the early postoperative period. Abdominal x-rays show dilated small bowel loops with air-fluid levels and absent or scant air in the colon. Laboratory testing may reveal leukocytosis. Decompression with a nasogastric or long intestinal tube is warranted, with the majority of cases responding to this conservative management. Persistent symptoms warrant surgical re-exploration.

24

Infections of the Genital Tract

Edward Tanner and Carolyn J. Alexander

1. A 19-year-old nulliparous woman presents to your office complaining of a yellow discharge for 3 days. She reports one new partner in the last 3 weeks with whom she has had unprotected intercourse. On speculum examination, a thick yellow discharge is present from the cervical os. No cervical motion tenderness, adnexal tenderness, or fullness are present. Gene probe is positive for *Chlamydia* and indeterminant for gonorrhea. Appropriate clinical evaluation and treatment would include all of the following, *except*:

A. Azithromycin 1 g PO, single dose

B. Azithromycin 1 g PO, single dose and ciprofloxacin 500 mg PO, single dose

C. Azithromycin 1 g PO, single dose and ceftriaxone 125 mg IM, single dose

D. Rapid plasma reagin (RPR), HIV, hepatitis B surface antigen titer, hepatitis C viral antibody titer

E. Notification of local health department and treatment of partner

A In addition to treatment for *Chlamydia trachomatis*, this patient requires treatment for presumed gonorrhea. The regimens mentioned in choices B and C would be recommended. The patient is also at higher risk of contracting other sexually transmitted diseases, including HIV, syphilis, hepatitis B, and C, as suggested in choice D. To avoid reinfection from the same partner and to limit community-wide spread of *Chlamydia,* the local health department should be notified immediately (choice E).

2. A 33-year-old gravida 3, para 1 0 1 1 presents for her first prenatal visit at 16 weeks gestational age by last menstrual period. Her past medical history is unremarkable and she experiences hives with penicillin. She delivered a full term infant 18 months ago. She reports no current problems, no history of sexually transmitted diseases. Her pelvic exam is within normal limits. Her prenatal labs are significant for a reactive RPR (titer 1:32). FTA-ABS is positive. Her HIV test is nonreactive. Appropriate management is:

A. No treatment is needed because of her low titer. Follow-up RPR yearly.

B. Treat her with doxycycline 100 mg PO twice daily for 2 weeks secondary to her penicillin allergy.

C. Treat her with erythromycin 500 mg PO every 6 hours for 3 weeks secondary to her penicillin allergy.

D. She should be treated with penicillin after undergoing desensitization.

E. Retreat her if RPR titer does not decrease to 1:1.

> **D** She is diagnosed with syphilis and needs to be treated. No alternatives to penicillin have been proven effective for treating syphilis in pregnant women. Pregnant women who have a history of penicillin allergy should be desensitized and treated with Benzathine penicillin **G** 2.4 million units IM in a single dose (choice D). Choices B and C are incorrect. Doxycycline should not be used during pregnancy and Erythromycin does not reliably cure an infected fetus. According to CDC guidelines, patients should be reexamined clinically and serologically 6 and 12 months after treatment; more frequently if follow-up is uncertain. Choice E is incorrect. If patients have persistent signs or symptoms or a sustained fourfold increase in RPR titer, they probably failed treatment or were reinfected and should be retreated and reevaluated for HIV infection. Failure of RPR titer to declined fourfold (i.e., 1:32 to 1:8) within 6 months after therapy for primary or secondary syphilis might indicate probable treatment failure. Because treatment failure may also suggest unrecognized CNS infection, many recommend CSF examination in such situations. HIV-infected patients should be reevaluated at 3, 6, 9, 12, and 24 months.

3. A 29-year-old para 3 0 0 3 presents to your office complaining of a slowly growing rubbery mass on her right labia. On examination, the lesion is soft, pedunculated, erythematous at its base, and mildly tender when touched. A small amount of dried blood can be seen at the base. This lesion is best characterized as follows:

A. The most likely cause of this lesion is the human papilloma virus, notably serotypes 16, 18, or 21.

B. The lesion should be excised because it is likely to lead to cancer in the future.

C. Biopsy is required to confirm diagnosis.

D. Pregnant and immunosuppressed patients are at higher risk of developing this lesion.

D The patient has a typical presentation of condyloma acuminatum, which is caused by the human papilloma virus (HPV). Serotypes consistent with condyloma include types 6 and 11 which are rarely malignant. Serotypes consistent with cervical dysplasia and carcinoma include types 16, 18, 31, and 33 which do not form condyloma. These soft, sessile, and/or pedunculated lesions can occur on any mucosal or dermal surface and vary widely in their size and formation. Biopsy is rarely necessary to establish diagnosis, although the clinician should take care to rule out the condyloma lata of primary syphilis (choice C). Although usually asymptomatic, these lesions may become painful if irritated, as has occurred in this case. These lesions may appear or worsen during pregnancy and immunocompromised states.

25

Ectopic Pregnancy

Melissa Yates and Jeremy King

1. A 25-year-old patient presents to the Emergency Department (ED), reporting right lower quadrant (RLQ) pain, nausea, and vomiting for 1 day. Vital signs are significant for a T 38.2, P 112, R 12, BP 100/75. Abdominal exam is notable for significant tenderness in the RLQ with hypoactive bowel sounds and voluntary guarding. On pelvic exam, no vaginal bleeding is present but moderate cervical motion tenderness. The patient reports that her last menstrual period was 2 weeks ago. A pregnancy test is negative, and the patient's WBC is 15,000. What would be the most appropriate course of action?

- **A.** No additional tests needed, symptoms will resolve in the next few days
- **B.** CT scan
- **C.** Ultrasound
- **D.** Admission for observation and pain control
- **E.** Assume that the patient has pelvic inflammatory disease (PID) and admit her for IV antibiotics

   B A CT scan would be the most reasonable test to order given this scenario. Although it would be prudent to obtain cervical cultures, the symptoms point more to a diagnosis of appendicitis than to PID. Ectopic pregnancy would be ruled out by the negative pregnancy test. Additional differential diagnoses could include ovarian torsion, PID, ruptured ovarian cyst, gastroenteritis, urinary tract infection, and a renal stone, though these are less likely.

2. A 19-year-old patient with a history of pelvic inflammatory disease (PID), 1 induced abortion, and 2 ectopic pregnancies presents to the ED, reporting left lower quadrant (LLQ) pain. Her pulse is 130 and her BP is 85/50. She is awake and conversant. On exam, her abdomen is markedly distended, and she demonstrates rebound tenderness and involuntary guarding with no bowel sounds. What would be the most appropriate next step in her workup?

A. Order a pelvic ultrasound.

B. Obtain a urine hCG, place two large bore IVs, type and cross match the patient for 2 units of blood, and call the OR for an emergency case.

C. Call a gynecology consult immediately.

D. Order a CBC, type and screen, and complete metabolic panel.

E. Obtain a full history and then order labs and a pelvic ultrasound.

B This scenario represents an unstable patient with what is most likely a ruptured ectopic pregnancy. Because she is tachycardic and has a surgical abdomen, she is an emergency surgical case. Time should not be taken to order a pelvic ultrasound or to await lab results. The gynecology surgical team should be alerted as soon as possible.

3. Which of the following is a radiographic sign of a normal intrauterine pregnancy?

A. Double decidual sign within the uterus

B. Free echogenic fluid in the pelvis

C. Increased blood flow to the adnexa

D. A cystic adnexal mass

E. Dilated and thick-walled fallopian tubes

A All of the other choices listed are radiographic signs of an ectopic pregnancy. To differentiate between a double decidual sign and a pseudosac, which can be seen with an ectopic pregnancy, is important. A pseudosac tends to be oval in shape and located in the center of the uterus, whereas the gestational sac of an intrauterine pregnancy tends to be more eccentrically located and has smooth borders. Doppler imaging can also be helpful in discerning a normal intrauterine pregnancy because there will be increased flow to the sac.

4. A patient is treated with methotrexate for a properly diagnosed ectopic pregnancy. Four days later, she presents with markedly increased abdominal pain. A repeat vaginal ultrasound is obtained, which demonstrates increased free fluid in the pelvis. What should the gynecology team do next?

A. Obtain repeat liver function studies.

B. Recheck the hCG level.

C. Give NSAIDS and closely monitor the patient for improvement.

D. Give a repeat dose of methotrexate.

E. Admit the patient for IV antibiotics.

C Increased abdominal pain at 4 days after injection is a common side effect of methotrexate treatment for ectopic pregnancy. Although patients should be closely monitored during these episodes of acute pain, most of the time the pain resolves with NSAIDS and does not require surgical intervention in a stable patient. Giving a repeat dose of methotrexate at this time would not be appropriate because the quantitative hCG is often higher at day 4 and should be rechecked at day 7 to determine whether an additional dose is warranted. This should be done only on the single dose protocol, if less than a 15% decline exists in hCG between days 1 and 7.

5. A patient is noted to have an ectopic pregnancy after an in-vitro fertilization procedure. Laparoscopic management is selected. During surgery, the ectopic is noted to be in a fallopian tube with a previously noted hydrosalpinx. What would be the appropriate management?

A. Perform a salpingostomy to preserve the tube.

B. Perform a salpingectomy to resect the hydrosalpinx.

C. Fimbriectomy and offer IVF

D. Perform bilateral salpingectomies because the patient had an ectopic with an IVF procedure, and the tubes must be damaged.

E. The patient should not have gone to surgery and should have been offered methotrexate to avoid adhesions caused by surgery.

B Salpingectomy is indicated in the situation of an ectopic in a known hydrosalpinx, because removal of the hydrosalpinx has been shown to increase the success rates of IVF in future cycles.

26

Chronic Pelvic Pain

Alexander Simopoulos

1. Although no universally accepted definition of *chronic pelvic pain* exists, which statement best characterizes chronic pelvic pain?

   A. Abdominal pain in any quadrant lasting for a duration of at least 4 to 6 months, generally attributed to a menstrual etiology

   B. Menstrual or nonmenstrual abdominal pain clinically apparent for 4 to 6 months without causing functional impairment

   C. Menstrual or nonmenstrual pain of at least 6 months duration, causing functional impairment, requiring medical or surgical treatment, and generally attributed to a disease process

   D. Menstrual or nonmenstrual pain of 6 or more months, below the umbilicus, severe enough to cause functional disability or require medical or surgical treatment

   D Choices A and B are incorrect because the duration of pain considered chronic by most clinicians is 6 months. Choice A is also incorrect because pain may be attributed to either a menstrual or a nonmenstrual etiology. Choice C is not correct because chronic pelvic pain is generally considered to be a symptom not a disease process.

2. A 45-year-old Caucasian woman presents to your office with a history of 7 months of cyclic bilateral lower abdominal pain. The patient gives you a detailed history, which includes a total abdominal hysterectomy with bilateral salpingo-oophorectomy for severe menorrhagia due to large uterine fibroids 3 years earlier at a resident teaching institution. She is not on hormone replacement therapy because she is concerned about her family history of breast cancer. She claims that she is lucky to not have experienced any menopausal symptoms. You order an ultrasound that confirms a surgically absent uterus and nonvisualization of the ovaries. The next most cost-effective step in confirming the diagnosis would be

A. Diagnostic laparoscopy

B. CT scan of the abdomen and pelvis

C. Exploratory laparotomy

D. Psychiatric referral

E. Order serum levels of follicle stimulating hormone (FSH) and estrogen.

E It seems very likely that patient is suffering from ovarian remnant syndrome. This syndrome is thought to be secondary to inadequate skeletonization of the infundibulopelvic ligaments and placement of clamps insufficiently lateral to include all ovarian tissue. Ordering the serum studies and finding premenopausal values would be highly suspicious for ovarian remnant syndrome. Further imaging (choice B) and laparoscopy (choice A) may not be helpful because ovarian remnants may require superovulation before surgery to help in identification. Although surgery and excision of ovarian tissue (choice C) will likely be necessary, this step is not the most cost-effective in diagnosis. Before referral for psychiatric evaluation (choice D), an organic etiology of the patient's pain should be pursued.

3. A 32-year-old patient presents to your clinic complaining of dyspareunia and lower abdominal pain. Upon further questioning, you are able to elicit that she has also been experiencing urinary frequency, urgency, and suprapubic pain, which subsides to a degree upon voiding. You suspect a diagnosis. Your next most appropriate step in the management of this patient is

A. Order a pelvic ultrasound.

B. Place intravesical dimethyl sulfoxide and oral pentosan polysulfate sodium.

C. Prescribe a trial of amitriptyline at bedtime and have the patient follow-up in 1 to 2 weeks.

D. Refer patient to the urology service.

E. Schedule a cystoscopy with hydrodistention.

E Accurate diagnosis of interstitial cystitis (IC) can be made only by cystoscopy and hydrodistention under anesthesia. The diagnosis can be confirmed by cystoscopic findings of glomerulations (Hunner's ulcers) as well as terminal hematuria. Ordering a pelvic ultrasound (choice A) would be useful if you suspected a possible ovarian or uterine etiology for the patient's pain. Although choices B and C are recognized therapies for IC, to first make a diagnosis is more important. In addition, hydrodistention in itself is a therapeutic modality. Referral to urology could conceivably occur based on the result of the cystoscopy, but this step is not the appropriate step for the practicing gynecologist.

4. A 46-year-old, distraught, obese woman presents to your office with complaints of severe menometrorrhagia, dysmenorrhea, and dyspareunia. You perform a physical exam of the patient, which reveals an enlarged, globular uterus. Given her history of these complaints over the last year, you also send a complete blood count that returns later in the afternoon with a hematocrit of 28. You have the patient return the following morning and you counsel her that the most appropriate management of your suspected diagnosis is

A. Trial of oral contraceptive pills (OCPs)

B. Nonsteroidal anti-inflammatory drugs (NSAIDs) at the time of menses

C. Diagnostic laparoscopy

D. Endometrial biopsy

E. Hysterectomy

F. Pelvic ultrasound

D It appears very likely that this patient is suffering from adenomyosis. Hysterectomy has been consistently shown to be successful in treating and controlling the symptoms associated with adenomyosis. However, given the patient's history of irregular bleeding, an evaluation is important for possible uterine pathology by performing a biopsy as well as a pap smear. OCPs (choice A) and NSAIDs (choice B) are more appropriate if a diagnosis of endometriosis is suspected. Diagnostic laparoscopy (choice C) may help visualize an enlarged globular uterus but is not reliable or cost-effective. Pelvic ultrasound (choice F) would be useful if fibroids were suspected but would do little to aid in the diagnosis of adenomyosis. MRI, however, can be used in the diagnosis.

27

Urogynecology and Reconstructive Pelvic Surgery

Francisco Rojas and Geoffrey W. Cundiff

1. A 39-year-old para 2-0-1-2, Caucasian woman comes to the clinic complaining of 1 year of worsening urinary urgency, frequency, and since 3 months ago, pelvic pain and occasional nocturia. She was evaluated recently in the emergency room, where complete blood count (CBC), urine culture, and transvaginal ultrasound were performed and were found to be within normal limits. Straight catheter urinalysis (UA) showed numerous red blood cells. Her past medical history is significant for two full-term spontaneous vaginal deliveries and mild asthma. She weighs 130 pounds, vital signs are normal, and the physical exam, including sterile speculum exam and bimanual pelvic exam, confirm an anteverted uterus and no adnexal masses. Today's UA shows 5 to 10 red blood cells. The most likely diagnosis is

A. Endometriosis

B. Persistent urinary tract infection

C. Painful bladder syndrome

D. Urethral diverticulum

E. Urge incontinence

C The International Continent Society (ICS) proposed a common language for lower urinary tract dysfunction in 2002. Painful bladder syndrome (PBS), formerly known as interstitial cystitis, is a chronic inflammatory condition with irritative voiding symptoms of urgency, frequency, pelvic, and lower urinary tract pain (70% cases). Dyspareunia, sleep disturbance, and incontinence may be present. This condition is characterized by a significant decrease in quality of life. Even though endometriosis may be associated with irritative urinary tract symptoms and pelvic pain, this condition is not the most likely diagnosis. Urinary tract infection is not probable, considering the duration of the symptoms and because the patient does not have fever or leukocytosis, and the urine culture was negative. Suburethral diverticulum is a fluid-filled mass along the anterior portion of the vagina that has a direct communication with the urethra. The cause is usually infection of a furuncle in a urethral gland. Other causes include birth trauma, instrumentation injury, and urethral stones. Suburethral diverticula are present in less than 3% of the general population. However, in patients with low urinary tract symptoms, the incidence could reach up to 40%. Patients usually have vague complaints. The most common symptoms are dysuria, suburethral mass, recurrent UTI, frequency, urgency, incontinence, and dribbling. The clinical presentation of this patient is not significant for incontinence.

2. The next step in her management is

A. Intravenous pyelogram (IVP)

B. Cystourethroscopy

C. Urodynamic studies

D. Tolterodine LA

E. Pelvic muscle exercises

B Cystourethroscopy is used to assess the anatomy of the lower urinary tract. It was considered the gold standard for diagnosis of IC. Positive findings consist of destructive changes of the mucosa (glomerulations, submucosal hemorrhages, ulcers); however, ulcers are seen in only advanced disease, and glomerulations can be observed in many normal individuals. Because cystoscopy has a 60% rate of underdiagnosis, this procedure is not recommended as a diagnostic test except to exclude other pathology, such as bladder cancer, tuberculosis, endometriosis, or stones. On the other hand, cystoscopy with hydrodistention is therapeutic in 20% to 30% of patients, with symptom relief for 3 to 6 months after distention. IVP provides anatomic and functional information about fistulas, duplicated or ectopic ureters, diverticulum, malignancy, stones, and obstructive uropathy, but is not the best option for this specific case. Urodynamic studies are a group of tests that assess the physiologic function of the bladder and evaluate bladder filling, urethral closure, and bladder emptying. They are especially useful in clinical scenarios that involve incontinence but cannot provide information about etiology of pain or hematuria. Pelvic muscle exercises are aimed at improving muscle tone. They can alleviate the symptoms of pelvic organ prolapse and urinary incontinence. Tolterodine and oxybutynin are anticholinergics and are first-line treatments for OAB, with acceptable side effects.

3. A 51-year-old Caucasian woman, para 2-1-1-3, has a long history of leaking of urine associated with episodes of coughing or sneezing when her bladder is full. Urodynamic studies failed to demonstrate involuntary detrusor contractions. Her physical exam is remarkable for a Q-tip test with the angle greater than 40 degrees and stage 1 pelvic organ prolapse. The most likely diagnosis is

A. Occult stress urinary incontinence

B. Intrinsic sphincter deficiency (ISD)

C. Mixed urinary incontinence

D. Stress urinary incontinence (SUI)

E. Overflow urinary incontinence

D Stress urinary incontinence (SUI) is the most common type of urinary incontinence among ambulatory incontinent women, accounting for 50% to 70% of cases. It occurs when the bladder neck and urethra fail to maintain a watertight seal under conditions of increased abdominal pressure, such as coughing, sneezing, laughing, walking, changing position, and even at rest in severe cases. This diagnosis excludes involuntary detrusor contraction as a cause of the leaking. Bladder capacity and postvoid residual are usually within normal limits. Traditionally, SUI was described as secondary to urethral hypermobility or intrinsic sphincter deficiency (ISD). However, the value of distinguishing between ISD and hypermobility has not been established. ISD is a condition characterized for abnormal sphincteric mechanism, which fails to close the UVJ. These patients are unable to maintain a watertight seal even at rest. They are often severely incontinent and can leak urine with minimal exertion. *Occult* or *reduced stress incontinence* are terms used to describe SUI, which is demonstrable only when the pelvic organ prolapse is reduced. Mixed incontinence is used to describe symptoms of both stress and urge incontinence. Overflow urinary incontinence is the continuous leaking as a consequence of urinary retention.

4. The most well-established surgery for this condition is

A. Anterior repair (Kelly's plication)

B. Needle procedures (Pereyra, Stamey)

C. Periurethral bulk injections

D. Retropubic urethropexy (Marshall-Marchetti-Krantz operation)

E. Retropubic bladder neck suspension (Burch)

> **E** In the Burch procedure, sutures are placed in the periurethral fascia lateral to and on each side of the bladder neck and proximal urethra (two sutures per side), and the UVJ is elevated by attaching the suture to Cooper's ligament with permanent sutures (tension-free). The 5-year success rate is 70% to 90%. The Burch procedure is the most well-established surgery for incontinence. The Burch procedure and slings, including TVT and TOT, appear equally efficacious. Also, operative complications and long-term voiding dysfunction were similar. The Marshall-Marchetti-Krantz procedure is similar to the Burch procedure, except that the sutures are attached to the symphysis pubis with risk for periostitis. Anterior repair has a 5-year success rate of 30% to 40% and can be useful in patients seeking minimal risks from surgery. Needle procedures have a poor long-term success rate and, in consequence, little role in current management. Periurethral bulk injections are best used in patients with urinary incontinence secondary to a poorly functioning urethral sphincter (ISD) or refractory incontinence in the absence of urethral hypermobility.

5. A 48-year-old woman, para 2-0-0-2, comes to the office describing symptoms of pressure and vaginal fullness. Occasionally, she has a sense of incomplete rectal and bladder emptying that improves with Valsalva maneuver or splinting. A sexual function questionnaire reveals dyspareunia and decreased libido. A complete physical exam confirms the presence of rectocele and cystocele, both 2 cm distal to the hymenal ring (+2). Based on the Pelvic Organ Prolapse Quantification (POPQ) system, the classification of this prolapse is

A. Stage 0

B. Stage 1

C. Stage 2

D. Stage 3

E. Stage 4

D See Figure 27-2 in the Manual text. In the POPQ system, stage 3 describes a pelvic organ prolapse when the lowest point is more than 1 cm distal to the hymenal ring but not completely prolapsed. Stage 0 is perfect support. Stage 1 implies that all points are more proximal than 1 cm to the hymenal ring. Stage 2 is used when the lowest point of the pelvic organ prolapse is between 1 cm proximal and 1 cm distal to the hymenal ring. Stage 4, or complete prolapse, has the lowest point equal to the total vaginal length (TVL).

28

Fertility Control: Contraception, Sterilization, and Abortion

Mary Ellen Pavone and Anne Burke

1. Which of the following methods of tubal ligation has the highest failure rate?

A. Laparoscopic bipolar coagulation

B. Laparoscopic unipolar coagulation

C. Postpartum partial salpingectomy

D. Laparoscopic silicone band application

A According to The Collaborative Review of Sterilization (CREST) study, which compared the long-term effectiveness of different sterilization procedures, spring clip application had the highest failure rate, followed by bipolar coagulation (see Table 28-2 in Manual).

2. Which of the following is true regarding emergency contraception?

A. The Copper IUD has been shown to be effective as an emergency contraceptive if placed 5 to 8 days after having unprotected intercourse.

B. The primary mechanism of action of Plan B is to disrupt implantation of the pregnancy.

C. Combined oral contraceptive pills have recently been shown to be more effective than progestin only pills for preventing pregnancy after unprotected intercourse.

D. Data show that emergency contraception must be initiated within 72 hours of unprotected intercourse to be effective.

A The Copper IUD is a very effective form of emergency contraception, with a pregnancy rate of 0.1% to 0.2% if inserted within 5 days of unprotected intercourse. If ovulation is known to have occurred 3 days or more after unprotected intercourse, the IUD may be inserted up to 8 days after intercourse. Choice B is incorrect because the primary mechanism of action of hormonal emergency contraception is to prevent pregnancy not disrupt an implanted pregnancy. Possibly, any change may affect the endometrium that would make implantation less likely, but recent studies show that this is not likely to occur. Choice C is incorrect because Plan B (progestin only) is both more effective and better tolerated (less nausea and vomiting) than combined oral contraceptives. Choice D is incorrect because, although it has been recommended to take the first dose within 72 hours of unprotected intercourse, evidence supports its effectiveness if used up to 120 hours after intercourse.

3. A 20-year-old G0 P0 comes to your office 3 months after starting combined oral contraceptives, complaining of having had several migraine headaches. While taking her history, you learn that her mother also suffers from occasional migraine headaches. However, this is a new problem for your patient. Your next action is to

   A. Ask the patient to follow up with neurology.

   B. Provide reassurance. Migraine headaches are a common side effect of combined oral contraceptive pills.

   C. Discontinue combined oral contraceptive use.

   D. Ask the patient to take continuous active pills and skip the placebo pills to see whether this lessens her migraine frequency.

   C Newly diagnosed migraine headaches should prompt the provider to discontinue combined oral contraceptive use. If the patient had a history of migraine headaches, the provider may consider continuous hormone administration.

4. Which of the following statements is true regarding medical termination of pregnancy with mifepristone and misoprostol?

   A. Medical termination can generally be performed up to 12 weeks of gestation.

   B. Side effects from the medications used to induce a medical abortion include bleeding and GI discomfort.

C. Women who undergo a medical termination of pregnancy do not need follow-up.

D. Methotrexate has higher efficacy and works faster than mifepristone.

B Evidence-based recommendations indicate that medical terminations with mifepristone and misoprostol can be performed up to 9 weeks' gestation. All women who undergo this procedure need follow-up. Mifepristone, not methotrexate, generally works faster, has higher efficacy, and is associated with fewer side effects.

5. All of the following statements are true regarding cervical dilation for pregnancy termination, *except:*

A. Osmotic dilators absorb cervical mucous and gradually enlarge the endocervical canal and soften the cervix.

B. Pratt, Hagar, or Denniston dilators can be used to mechanically dilate the cervix.

C. Methotrexate can be used preoperatively to soften the cervix.

D. Very early pregnancies may not require additional cervical dilation.

C Misoprostol and mifepristone, but not methotrexate, can be used preoperatively to soften and dilate the cervix.

29

Domestic Violence and Sexual Assault

Jacqueline Baselice

1. Which of the following statements regarding domestic violence and sexual assault is false?

A. Nearly 25% of women in the United States will be abused by a current or former partner in their lifetime.

B. Gay and lesbian relationships have a decreased incidence of abuse.

C. More than 75% of adolescent rapes are committed by an acquaintance.

D. One in four women will experience a sexual act without consent during their college years.

B Lesbian relationships have the same frequency of abuse as heterosexual relationships, and screening all patients for domestic violence is important regardless of their sexual orientation.

2. After a patient is evaluated for rape, the provider should follow up with the patient

A. In 1 to 2 weeks for psychological evaluation and repeat pregnancy test

B. In 4 weeks for repeat hepatitis B vaccine, collections of cultures for test of cure, and repeat pregnancy test

C. In 3 to 6 months for repeat HIV, hepatitis B, and syphilis

D. All of the above

D Close follow-up is very important with a patient who is a victim of rape. When the patient first presents, she is treated presumptively for STDS, given ceftriaxone, and doxycycline or azithromycin to cover gonorrhea and *Chlamydia,* respectively. She should also be given the hepatitis B vaccine if she has not already received it. At each of these visits, she should be screened for rape-trauma syndrome, which may include feelings of anger, fear, shame, nightmares, and other symptoms of posttraumatic stress syndrome.

3. In providing adolescents with counseling for preventing sexual assault, the following should be stressed, *except:*

   A. Do not leave parties with someone whom you do not know well.

   B. Be aware of your surroundings at all times and avoid situations that may put you at risk.

   C. Dress conservatively so as to not send the wrong message to others.

   D. Set sexual limits and insist that your partner honor them.

   C Counseling adolescents should be empowering them to take an active role in preventing sexual assault, and fashion decisions do not play a role. Adolescents should be aware that no one should ever be forced or pressured to engage in unwanted sexual activity, and it does not matter what one is wearing.

4. A 16-year-old gravida 1, para 0 at 34$^{1}/_{7}$ weeks' gestation presents to Labor and Delivery with her boyfriend after she fell on her abdomen at home. She complains of abdominal pain since the accident. While conducting the history and physical, doing all of the following is important, *except:*

   A. Determine the cause of the fall.

   B. Keep the boyfriend in the room, because she says that he was there to help her off the ground. He may be able to give more history about how she fell.

   C. Ask if she is having any vaginal bleeding, contractions, or feeling the baby move.

   D. Do a full physical exam, looking for other areas with evidence of trauma.

B Interviewing the patient in private is important to allow for full disclosure of events and to allow the patient to feel safe. The batterer will often accompany the victim to appointments and wants to stay close at hand to monitor what she says to the physician. While doing the physical, if there are other signs of abuse, they should be documented as well, such as other bruises or scars. In determining the cause of the fall, one should ask if domestic violence is a possibility. Routinely asking patients about domestic violence significantly increases its detection.

5. After the boyfriend leaves, the patient denies that she is a victim of domestic abuse. Upon reviewing her chart, you find that she has been to Labor and Delivery multiple times for falls, headaches, and back pain. You readdress the issue with the patient, and she confides to you that she has been abused during this pregnancy and is ready to make a change for the safety of her fetus. A successful exit plan should include

   A. Falsified birth certificate and drivers license so she cannot be tracked down by the abuser.

   B. Deciding upon a plan of exactly where to go, regardless of the time, day, or night.

   C. Having a change of clothes packed for herself under the bed, so she can grab it in a hurry.

   D. Gradually taking small amounts of cash from her partner without him knowing, so she will have enough money when she leaves.

   B In empowering a victim of domestic violence, reviewing an exit plan with her is important. It should include having a change of clothes and an extra set of house and car keys in a suitcase, at a friend or neighbor's house, as well as a checkbook, cash, or savings account book kept with that designated person. Also, identification papers should be kept available for possible financial assistance.

30

Pediatric Gynecology

Dayna Finkenzeller

1. A mother presents to the Emergency Department with her 2-year-old daughter who has been complaining of "hurting 'down there' when I pee." Her mother notes that she has also been increasingly irritable at home over the past few days. She reports her daughter has otherwise been healthy in the past. Physical exam and vital signs are remarkable for a low grade temperature of 99.1°F and mild suprapubic tenderness. No evidence of rebound, guarding, or CVA tenderness is present, and external pelvic exam is unremarkable. Urinalysis is obtained and is notable for 25 to 30 white blood cells, 5 to 10 red blood cells, and 2 to 3 epithelial cells, with positive leukocyte esterase and positive nitrites. Urine culture has been sent. Your next step in management is

A. Ciprofloxacin, 7-day course; follow up for worsening symptoms

B. Bactrim, 7-day course; follow up for worsening symptoms

C. Send the patient home and wait for urine culture results.

D. Ciprofloxacin, 7-day treatment course followed by maintenance suppression therapy. If urine culture results are positive, obtain a renal ultrasound or voiding cystourethrogram.

E. Bactrim, 7-day treatment course followed by maintenance suppression therapy. If urine culture results are positive, obtain a renal ultrasound or voiding cystourethrogram.

E Choices A and D are incorrect because fluoroquinolones should be avoided in this age group secondary to the risks of cartilage toxicity. Ciprofloxacin is not FDA approved in children under age 18, except in cases of anthrax or complicated urinary tract infections. Choices B and C are incorrect because the first diagnosed UTI in a child needs to be further evaluated with radiographic imaging. A complete radiographic evaluation is indicated in children with UTI and fever, girls under age 3 with a UTI, and children with UTI who do not respond to therapy. Reinfection occurs within 18 months in 40% to 60% of all children. Detection of anatomic irregularities associated with vesicoureteral reflux (VUR) can result in more aggressive management to help prevent renal scarring. The nephropathy that results from renal scarring is the most common disorder leading to hypertension in children.

2. A 2-year-old girl is referred to your office by her pediatrician, with a vaginal mass noted on annual exam. On pelvic examination, you note a polypoid mass protruding from the vagina that appears friable and bleeds easily with manipulation. You are able to take a small biopsy of the mass in your office and pathology demonstrates sarcoma botryoides. Your next step is to

A. Obtain a CT scan and chest x-ray.

B. Consent the patient and her mother to take the patient to the operating room for excision of the polypoid mass under general endotracheal anesthesia.

C. Consult medical oncology to initiate an appropriate chemotherapeutic regimen.

D. Consult radiation oncology to initiate whole pelvic irradiation.

A Sarcoma botryoides is the most common malignant tumor of the genital tract in girls. It is characteristically fast-growing, aggressive, and in 90% of cases occurs before age 5, with a peak incidence at age 2. This tumor arises in the submucosa of the vagina then penetrates through, creating a hallmark polypoid mass passing from the vagina, vulva, or urethra. Patients often present with vaginal bleeding and abdominal pain. The first step in management is to stage with chest x-ray and CT scan. If the mass is resectable, chemotherapy should be initiated followed by radical hysterectomy and vaginectomy. If the lesion is not resectable, radiotherapy should be used as first-line treatment. Close follow-up is required because sarcoma botryoides tend to recur locally.

3. A 17-year-old girl presents to your office with primary amenorrhea, and she is not yet sexually active. On exam, breasts are consistent with Tanner stage V development, but she has only scant pubic and axillary hair. On pelvic examination, her vagina ends in a blind pouch and you obtain a pelvic ultrasound that reveals absence of a uterus, cervix, and fallopian tubes, and the presence of bilateral masses that appear to have descended through the inguinal canal. Your next step in management is to

A. Obtain a CT or MRI.

B. Initiate estrogen therapy.

C. Refer the patient to a psychologist for counseling and coping mechanisms.

D. Schedule the patient for surgical resection of the bilateral pelvic masses.

D The clinical scenario described is consistent with a male feminization syndrome in which genetic males (XY) undergo feminization related to androgen insensitivity. Complete androgen insensitivity, or "testicular feminization," is transmitted in a maternal X-linked recessive fashion. In this condition, androgen presence is unable to induce the Wolffian duct to mature and, as a result, seminal vesicles, vas deferens, and epididymis do not form. Antimüllerian duct hormone is present so müllerian duct formation remains inhibited such that uterus, cervix, and fallopian tubes do not form either. The resulting phenotype is female with a vagina derived from the urogenital sinus that ends in a blind pouch and testes that often descend through the inguinal canal.

Patients often present with primary amenorrhea, Tanner stage V breast development and scant axillary and pubic hair. Gonadectomy is strongly recommended secondary to an increased incidence of malignancy.

4. A worried mother has brought her 3-year-old daughter to your office because she has noticed that her daughter has been developing breast buds over the past 2 months. She reports that her daughter has no significant past medical history and takes no medications. On examination, the child has Tanner stage IV breast development with no evidence of axillary or pubic hair. External genitalia appear within normal limits. You obtain a pelvic ultrasound that reveals a normal prepubertal uterus and plain films demonstrate normal bone age for a 3-year-old child. You counsel the child's mother by informing her that

A. Her child needs immediate biopsy of her breast tissue and evaluation by a surgical oncologist.

B. Her child needs a breast biopsy.

C. Her child needs a mammogram.

D. This condition is often temporary and will often resolve on its own. She will need to follow up in 3 to 4 months.

D Premature thelarche is a condition in which bilateral breast development occurs without other signs of sexual maturation in girls before age of 8. It most commonly occurs by age 2 and is rare after age 4. The etiology behind premature thelarche is unclear, but an exogenous estrogen source must be excluded. Premature thelarche is not known to be associated with central nervous system pathology and is not known to be a familial condition. The mechanism is thought to be related to a temporary activation of the hypothalamic-pituitary-gonadal axis with increased FSH secretion. On initial workup, precocious puberty must be ruled out. Bone age can be determined with radiographic imaging and should be within normal range in premature thelarche and advanced in precocious puberty. Pelvic sonography should demonstrate a normal prepubertal uterus.

Plasma estrogen levels may be mildly elevated, but dramatic elevations suggest another etiology. Stimulated responses of LH and FSH may be obtained and are generally both elevated in precocious puberty, whereas only stimulated FSH is elevated in premature thelarche. Also, review recently used medications and topical creams as application of topical conjugated estrogens, such as Premarin, for longer than 2 to 3 weeks may result in breast changes. In idiopathic cases, a regression in breast enlargement often occurs after a few months but may persist for several years. In approximately 50% of patients, breast development can last 3 to 5 years.

31

Infertility and Assisted Reproductive Technologies

Eli A. Rybak and Edward E. Wallach

1. A couple presents for an initial infertility workup. The woman is a 39-year-old nullipara; her 40-year-old husband underwent chemotherapy for a childhood leukemia. They report 12 months of well-timed intercourse based on positive home urinary LH monitoring. Which of the following statements regarding the infertility evaluation for this couple is true?

   A. Inability to achieve pregnancy after 12 months of well-timed intercourse is unsurprising; referral to an infertility specialist is only warranted after 36 months of unsuccessful attempts at conception.

   B. Given the husband's history, the couple should pursue adoption or artificial insemination with donor sperm.

   C. Ovulatory dysfunction has been excluded given the positive urinary LH testing.

   D. Given the advanced reproductive age of the woman, this couple should be referred directly to IVF.

   E. If the semen analysis demonstrates a zoospermia, this couple may benefit from IVF with ICSI.

   E The American Society for Reproductive Medicine defines infertility as a disease and recommends, "The duration of the failure to conceive should be twelve or more months before an investigation is undertaken unless medical history and physical findings dictate earlier evaluation and treatment" (Practice Committee Opinion, March 27, 1993).

   The cumulative odds of pregnancy after 12 months of well-timed intercourse reach 85%. Patients should be advised of the epidemiologic studies demonstrating that the monthly fertile window occurs during the 6-day interval approaching the moment of ovulation. This couple warrants a comprehensive infertility evaluation; choice A is false. Given the advanced reproductive age of the woman, many authorities would recommend intervention even after only 6 months of futile attempts at conception. A precipitous drop occurs in pregnancy rates after age 35. This decline reflects the diminished ovarian reserve resulting from acceleration in oocyte aging and atresia as a woman approaches the perimenopause. Often, such women demonstrate elevated day 3 serum FSH levels or exaggerated FSH responses to the clomiphene challenge test. These findings portend a reduced likelihood of successful ovarian hyperstimulation and IVF. Accordingly, choice D is false: Ovarian reserve should be assessed before referral for assisted reproduction. Women found to have elevated FSH levels can be encouraged to consider using donor eggs. Finally, the likelihood of male factor infertility in this scenario mandates a semen analysis and male factor workup before precipitous enrollment in IVF.

Advances in intracytoplasmic sperm injection (ICSI) have enabled men with severe male factor infertility to bear genetically related offspring. The correct answer is choice E; in the likely scenario of abnormal semen parameters from this patient, recourse to IVF with ICSI should prove beneficial. Recourse to adoption or donor sperm should not be automatic; choice B is false.

Finally, one should not assume that ovulation is conclusively confirmed by a positive urinary LH assay. As noted in the text, over 7% of positive results are false. The midluteal progesterone level (concentrations exceeding 3.0 ng/mL between days 19 and 23) should remain the gold standard for confirmation of ovulation; choice C is therefore false.

2. Essential components of the infertility evaluation for this couple include all of the following tests, *except*:

   A. Hysterosalpingogram

   B. Cycle day 2 or 3 serum FSH

   C. Testicular biopsy

D. Endometrial biopsy

E. Semen analysis

D Although this couple's history suggests infertility stemming from male factor and/or depleted ovarian reserve, the initial evaluation should attempt exclusion of other causes of infertility. Over 30% of couples who present for assisted reproduction are diagnosed with multiple causes for their infertility. This couple's evaluation, for example, may well reveal both adequate ovarian reserve and normal semen parameters. A hysterosalpingogram (HSG) that offers insight into uterine or tubal structural abnormalities may mandate reparative surgery before initiation of ART. Moreover, despite potentially adequate ovarian reserve, the woman may have occult ovulatory dysfunction that could be detected by a progesterone assessment in the midluteal phase or late luteal phase endometrial biopsy. Semen analysis is not indicated (D).

3. Which of the following statements regarding ICSI is true?

A. ICSI has been shown to be as safe a procedure to resulting offspring as IVF.

B. Safety concerns confronting ICSI exceed those of IVF.

C. ICSI must be used only in the presence of severe male factor infertility.

D. Patients with unexplained infertility benefit from proceeding directly to ICSI.

E. Performing ICSI during IVF for male factor infertility has been associated with success rates exceeding those of IVF for tubal factor infertility

B ICSI involves IVF after micromanipulation of a single spermatozoon and oocyte. First performed in 1992, this procedure has dramatically reduced the reliance upon donor sperm among men with obstructive and nonobstructive azoospermia. Although it remains an acceptably safe procedure, ICSI poses safety concerns exceeding those of routine IVF. Choice A is false; choice B is the correct response. ICSI has been attributed to a significant increase in sex and autosomal chromosome abnormalities. Moreover, evidence links ICSI to various imprinting disorders. In cases of hereditary male infertility, ICSI enables the potential vertical transmission of this infertility to resulting male offspring.

Choices D and E are incorrect. Although ICSI for male factor infertility has dramatically increased the IVF success rates for such individuals, these success rates still lag behind those of IVF performed for nonmale factor infertility. This—and because ICSI presents additional health concerns—renders inappropriate any direct referral of couples with unexplained infertility to ICSI. Instead, unexplained infertility can be empirically treated by COH plus either intrauterine insemination or IVF. ICSI, however, can be indicated in circumstances that do not involve severe male factor infertility: Assisted reproduction for HIV serodiscordant couples, for example, relies on ICSI to reduce the likelihood of viral transmission. Additionally, IVF cycles during PGD typically use ICSI to minimize the chance of contamination from multiple spermatozoa embedded in the zona pellucida. Choice C is therefore false.

4. A couple—both partners age 28 and otherwise healthy—has been diagnosed with ovulatory dysfunction and tubal factor infertility. Controlled ovarian hyperstimulation (COH) has been initiated for IVF, using recombinant FSH and a GnRH agonist in a luteal phase protocol.

Benefits associated with the adjunctive use of GnRH agonists in the COH preceding IVF include all of the following, *except*:

A. Reduced requirements for gonadotropins

B. Increased number and quality of oocytes recovered per cycle

C. Increased fertilization and pregnancy rate

D. Reduced incidence of premature LH surge

E. Increased synchronization of recovered oocytes

A Whether the flare-up or luteal phase protocol is used, GnRH agonist downregulation reduces the premature luteinization and LH surges that precipitate cycle cancellations. Additionally, this adjunctive use of GnRH agonists increases the quantity, quality, and synchronization of recruited follicles. Resulting fertilization, pregnancy, and live birth rates are improved. Choices B, C, D, and E all reflect benefits associated with GnRH agonist use. Choice A is false and, thus, is the correct answer. Drawbacks of GnRH agonist use include *increased* gonadotropin requirements given the downregulation of the gonadotropin receptor and a potential risk for excessive estradiol levels and development of the ovarian hyperstimulation syndrome.

5. During COH, the woman complains of bloating, shortness of breath, and negligible urine output over the preceding 24-hour period. Proper management entails all of the following, *except*:

  A. Admission for inpatient monitoring of fluid status, renal, and pulmonary function

  B. Cycle cancellation

  C. Avoiding embryo transfer and converting to a cryopreservation cycle

  D. Prompt administration of hCG to trigger oocyte maturation

  E. Minimizing the dose of gonadotropins in subsequent cycles of COH

  D The ovarian hyperstimulation syndrome (OHSS) is an iatrogenic disorder caused by excessive responses to COH. Typically self-limiting and mild in severity, the OHSS can also manifest itself as a life-threatening disorder characterized by significant third-spacing, edema, weight gain, ascites, hydrothorax, ARDS, hypercoagulability and thrombosis, hemoconcentration, electrolyte derangement, and organ failure. The Golan classification scheme marshals clinical symptomatology, findings at ultrasonography, and laboratory results to stratify OHSS into various stages and grades of severity. Mild cases can be managed in the outpatient setting. Patients should be carefully counseled regarding the risks of ovarian torsion and the need to preserve intravascular fluid volume and electrolyte balance. Sports drinks are recommended in this regard. Severe cases of OHSS warrant hospitalization. Inpatient monitoring and intervention is calibrated to the severity and exact clinical manifestations of the particular case.

  Prevention techniques involve both "evasive" action and adjustments to future cycles of COH. During the actual cycle involving OHSS, consideration should be given to lowering or withholding the hCG dose administered for final oocyte maturation. Known as coasting, the administration of hCG is delayed until estradiol levels plateau over a defined course of time. Alternatively, the complete withholding of hCG will necessitate in vitro maturation of the aspirated oocytes. In severe cases, the cycle may be canceled altogether. Consideration should be given to cryopreserving any embryos attained should egg retrieval take place. Future cycles of COH should use the minimal amount of gonadotropin doses possible, and consideration should be given to substituting a GnRH antagonist for the GnRH agonist used during downregulation.

Choices A, B, C, and E represent appropriate management decisions. Choice D is the correct answer; hCG should not be given at this point, or at all, when confronted by impending OHSS. The administration of hCG during COH remains a major trigger for OHSS development.

6. Which statement regarding COH and IVF is true?

A. GnRH agonists are superior to GnRH antagonists with regards to preventing both premature LH surges and the OHSS.

B. Follicular recruitment is crucial; the more embryos transferred, the higher the live birth per transfer rate.

C. A patient with pelvic pain and vaginal bleeding after IVF/embryo transfer should be treated as having an ectopic pregnancy unless an intrauterine pregnancy can be confirmed.

D. COH using recombinant FSH affords significantly higher pregnancy rates than COH using hMG.

E. IVF cycles performed for sibling HLA matching via PGD warrant maximal follicular recruitment during COH.

E Choices A through D are false, thus choice E is the correct answer. GnRH antagonists provide comparable efficacy to GnRH agonist protocols, with several important advantages. Antagonists minimize gonadotropin doses by shortening the COH treatment interval. Moreover, they reduce the incidence of both premature LH surges and OHSS.

High-order embryo transfer does not lead to an increased live birth rate. Particularly among younger women, the highest live birth success rates are achieved when only two embryos are transferred. Higher-order embryo transfers do increase the rate of triplet pregnancies and should be avoided, which is reflected in the recently promulgated ASRM practice guidelines on embryo transfer.

Choice C expresses a potentially dangerous misnomer. Generally speaking, the presence of an intrauterine pregnancy (IUP) excludes the presence of a coexisting ectopic pregnancy in clinical decision making. The underlying rationale stems from the remote incidence of heterotopic pregnancy in the general population— estimates run as low as 1 in 30,000. Among women having undergone assisted reproduction, however, the incidence of heterotopic pregnancy can reach 1%. The confirmation of an IUP, accordingly, does not necessarily exclude a coexisting ectopic pregnancy.

The component of LH found in human menopausal gonadotropins (hMG, trade names Humegon and Repronex) has been thought to limit the effectiveness of COH. Efforts at purifying the FSH used for COH motivated the development of pure urinary FSH (Metrodin), ultrapure FSH (Fertinex), and then recombinant FSH (Gonal F, Follistim, and Puregon). Current data, however, have not conclusively demonstrated that recombinant FSH offers superior pregnancy success rates.

Choice E is true. When PGD is used for both hereditary disease prevention and sibling HLA matching, maximal follicular recruitment is critical. A quick review of Mendelian calculations indicates why: For an autosomal recessive disorder, three-fourths of embryos are statistically expected to be unaffected and, thus, transferable. In contrast, only one-fourth of embryos are expected to be HLA compatible to an older sibling. By multiplying these independently assorting probabilities, only three-sixteenths of embryos should be both unaffected from the hereditary disorder and HLA-compatible. Successful PGD in this case, therefore, relies upon a successful COH, with a large number of recruited follicles.

32

Recurrent Pregnancy Loss

Kristy Ruis and Kristiina Altman

1. Which of the following uterine anomalies is most commonly associated with recurrent pregnancy loss?

   A. Uterine synechiae

   B. Uterine didelphys

   C. Septate uterus

   D. Bicornuate uterus

   C Uterine malformations are noted in 12% to 15% of women who experience recurrent pregnancy loss. Congenital anomalies involve developmental defects involving the Müllerian duct, including septate, bicornuate, unicornuate, and didelphic uteri. Spontaneous pregnancy losses associated with anatomic causes occur most commonly in the second trimester; however, earlier losses can occur. The most common congenital malformation associated with recurrent pregnancy loss is septate uterus. Hysteroscopic repair by resection of the septum has been associated with improved pregnancy outcomes.

2. A 31-year-old para 0040 presents for preconception counseling. She has a history of four spontaneous abortions in the first trimester. Chromosomal analysis performed on all the abortuses were found to be normal. The patient reveals in her family history that her mother had a deep venous thrombosis at age 35. Which of the following laboratory tests might be useful in the evaluation of this patient?

   A. Factor V Leiden

   B. Prothrombin G20210A mutation

C. Antithrombin III

D. Methylenetetrahydrofolate reductase

E. Protein C deficiency

F. Protein S deficiency

G. Homocysteine level

H. All of the above

H Factor V Leiden deficiency, prothrombin G20210A mutation, antithrombin III deficiency, methylenetetrahydrofolate reductase deficiency, protein C deficiency, protein C resistance, protein S deficiency, and hyperhomocysteinemia are all associated with thrombus formation and have been associated with an increased risk of fetal loss. Although the risk of fetal loss is higher throughout pregnancy, the risk appears to be highest in the second and third trimesters. Thrombosis of spiral arteries and the associated uteroplacental vascular abnormalities can result in late fetal demise. The most common of the inherited disorders are Factor V Leiden deficiency and Prothrombin mutation. Screening for thrombophilias should be performed. Evidence for antithrombotic therapy in treating recurrent pregnancy loss and thrombophilia is limited. Some preliminary data have suggested that treatment with low molecular weight heparin may improve pregnancy outcome.

3. A 41-year-old woman presents for her first prenatal visit at 6 weeks' gestation. Based on her age, what is the likelihood that she will experience a spontaneous pregnancy loss?

A. 15%

B. 30%

C. 50%

D. 75%

D Ten percent to 15% of pregnancies result in first and early second-trimester losses, and 80% of all spontaneous losses will occur during the first trimester. One percent of all reproductive age women will experience recurrent pregnancy loss. The risk of spontaneous loss increases with age. In women age 40 and older, the spontaneous loss rate is around 75%.

4. Most commonly, early pregnancy losses are related to which of the following?

A. Turner's syndrome (45X)

B. Autosomal trisomies

C. Parental balanced translocations

D. Parental mosaicism

B Seventy percent of early pregnancy losses are related to chromosomal abnormalities of the fetus. The most frequent abnormalities are autosomal trisomies, most commonly 13, 16, 18, 21, and 22. 45X is the second most common abnormality. If aneuploidy is diagnosed in the first fetal loss, chromosomal abnormalities are found approximately 70% of the time in recurrent losses. When parental karyotyping is performed, one partner in 3% to 8% of couples will be diagnosed with a chromosomal abnormality, most commonly a balanced translocation. A small percentage of abnormal parental karyotypes includes inversions or mosaicisms.

33

Uterine Leiomyomas

Jennifer Kulp and John Griffith

1. A 44-year-old woman comes to your office for follow-up for a newly diagnosed fibroid uterus. She asks you how common fibroids are. Approximately what percentage do you tell her that fibroids are present in women?

   A. 1%
   B. 10% to 15%
   C. 20% to 50%
   D. 75%

   C Uterine leiomyomas are the most common pelvic tumors in women. They have traditionally been described as present in 20% of women over age 35, but their presence in 50% of postmortem examinations indicates a much higher frequency.

2. A 50-year-old woman with known fibroids comes to your office. She complains of significant cramping, heavy bleeding, and pelvic pressure related to the fibroids. She is tired of these symptoms and tells you that she desires a hysterectomy. She also complains of occasional hot flashes. On physical exam, you note a 14-week-sized uterus that is comparable in size from the previous year. In counseling your patient, you tell her that

   A. In greater than half of cases, leiomyomas will increase in size in women ages 50 to 60.
   B. With the onset of menopause, leiomyomas tend to regress in volume.
   C. Her symptoms are unrelated to her fibroids.

D. A hysterectomy during the perimenopausal period is recommended because it will ease her transition to menopause.

B The growth of uterine leiomyomas is clearly related to their exposure to circulating estrogen. These tumors are most prominent and demonstrate maximal growth during the reproductive years, when ovarian estrogen secretion is maximal. With the onset of menopause, leiomyomas tend to regress in volume. Whenever leiomyomas grow after menopause, malignancy must be seriously considered. When women with fibroids experience symptoms related to their fibroids, the most common are pain, pressure, and menorrhagia. As leiomyomas tend to become smaller after menopause, most patients in perimenopause will benefit from expectant management of fibroids.

3. A 35-year-old, gravida 1, para 1-0-0-1, African American woman presents to your office for a routine gynecologic exam. She uses condoms for contraception, has never had an abnormal pap smear, and has no complaints today. Her last gynecologic visit was 3 years ago. On physical exam, you note an approximately 16-week-sized uterus, irregular in shape. Her urine pregnancy test is negative. To work up your physical exam findings you order

A. Hysterosalpingography (HSG)

B. Sonohysterography

C. Abdominal/transvaginal ultrasound

D. Magnetic resonance imaging (MRI)

C Abdominal/transvaginal ultrasound. Ultrasound is a good method for detecting the presence of fibroids and is also useful for following their growth. A hysterosalpingogram can identify fibroids that are impinging on the uterine cavity and is a useful part of an infertility workup. It also evaluates the patency of fallopian tubes. Likewise, sonohysterography, in which ultrasound is used to evaluate the uterus after saline is infused into the uterine cavity, is useful for detecting fibroids that may be distorting the uterine cavity. Neither of these methods are good at detecting the precise location of fibroids. MRI is useful for defining the exact location and size of fibroids. However, the expense prevents it from being used routinely to diagnose fibroids. MRI is more commonly used for evaluation before procedures, such as uterine artery embolization.

4. A 30-year-old woman who has never been pregnant presents to your office after having a newly diagnosed fibroid uterus. She is asymptomatic, and the fibroids were noted on a routine exam. She subsequently had an ultrasound. The ultrasound showed the overall uterine size to be approximately 14 cm with multiple fibroids. The largest fibroids are a 2 × 2 cm anterior fibroid and a 3 × 2 cm posterior fibroid. She asks you about treatment for her fibroids. You recommend

   A. Observation with a repeat ultrasound in 6 to 8 weeks

   B. A course of gonadotropin-releasing hormone analogs

   C. Myomectomy

   D. Hysterectomy

   E. Uterine artery embolization (UAE)

   A For a patient with newly diagnosed, small, asymptomatic fibroids, observation is the best management. Physical and ultrasonographic examinations should be performed initially and repeated in 6 to 8 weeks to document size and growth pattern. If growth is stable, the patient may be followed at 3- to 4-month intervals. In patients who have symptomatic fibroids, a trial of gonadotropin-releasing hormone analogs (GnRHa) may be indicated. GnRHa have been used successfully to achieve hypoestrogenism in various estrogen-dependent conditions. Reduction in tumor size of approximately 50% on average has been observed with the use of GnRHa over a 3-month course of treatment. These agents are useful as a conservative therapy or as an adjunct to surgical treatment. Myomectomy is the procedure of choice for a solitary pedunculated leiomyoma. Other indications for a myomectomy include interference with fertility or predisposition to repeated pregnancy loss due to the nature or location of leiomyomas. These do not apply to this patient, and therefore she would not be a candidate for a myomectomy. Hysterectomy is a definitive therapy for fibroids but is not considered first-line therapy. UAE is a procedure that works by occluding the uterine artery, which decreases the blood supply to the uterus and, ultimately, to the leiomyoma. The procedure is performed by placing a catheter into the femoral artery and accessing the hypogastric arteries, which are then occluded by substances, such as Gelfoam, absolute alcohol, or Ivalon particles (polyvinyl alcohol). It would not be the correct management for a patient with newly diagnosed, small fibroids.

34

Endometriosis

Melissa Yates and Nikos Vlahos

1. Which of the following is *not* evidence cited to support Sampson's theory regarding the cause of endometriosis?

A. Retrograde menstruation has been visualized during laparoscopy.

B. Endometriosis lesions are most commonly found in the dependent portions of the pelvis.

C. Elevated levels of IL-6 and TNF-α have been found in the peritoneal fluid of endometriosis patients.

D. Endometriosis has been seen in patients with obstruction to outward menstrual flow.

E. Endometriosis increased in women with longer duration of menstrual flow.

C All of the answers, except C, are supported by Sampson's theory of retrograde menstruation. Although inflammatory factors have been found in the peritoneal fluid of patients with endometriosis, they are not one of the supporting findings specific to Sampson's theory. IL-6 and TNF-α fit into the theory that many specific immunologic factors may play into the pathogenesis of endometriosis.

2. A 25-year-old para 0 presents to the office, reporting severe dysmenorrhea, which starts approximately 2 days before the onset of menses and continues throughout her period. She describes the pain as being central in location and also reports that she experienced dyspareunia the week before her period. She feels that these symptoms are becoming worse over time.

What would be the best way to diagnose the cause of this patient's pelvic pain?

A. Place the patient on continuous combined oral contraceptives to see whether the symptoms improve.

B. Immediately start the patient on a 6-month course of Lupron.

C. Obtain a pelvic ultrasound.

D. Schedule the patient for a diagnostic laparoscopy with possible tissue biopsies.

E. Perform a pelvic exam under anesthesia to feel for adhesions and/or nodularity.

> **D** The gold standard for diagnosing endometriosis is to perform a diagnostic laparoscopy and to obtain a tissue biopsy to confirm endometriosis. A patient with these symptoms may be started on combined oral contraceptives, but the actual diagnosis of endometriosis cannot be made. A patient should not be started on Lupron without an official diagnosis secondary to the side-effect profile. A pelvic ultrasound may not be helpful because, though it may be able to diagnose endometriomas, this technique is not able to visualize small areas of peritoneal lesions and/or adhesions. A pelvic exam under anesthesia may be helpful, but many patients with endometriosis do not have uterosacral nodularity or palpable adhesions.

3. When treating a patient for endometriosis with GnRH agonists, such as Lupron, what is an important modality to also include?

A. Fosamax to promote bone health.

B. Add-back combined hormonal replacement therapy.

C. No additional treatment should be given during that time.

D. Monthly bone density studies.

E. Premarin vaginal cream to reduce vaginal dryness.

> **B** Add-back combined hormone replacement therapy has been shown to improve both vasomotor symptoms and bone mineral density loss for patients who are being treated with GnRH agonists for endometriosis. Using add-back therapy has not been shown to decrease overall pain improvement from endometriosis. The most often recommended regimen is a daily conjugated estrogen 0.625 mg, with 2.5 mg of medroxyprogesterone acetate.

4. A 49-year-old patient presents with a long history of endometriosis, diagnosed by a biopsy performed during laparoscopy, desires a hysterectomy. She wishes to leave at least
one ovary in place, assuming they appear to be visually without endometriosis or additional pathology. What is the patient's risk of recurrent symptoms, if an ovary is left in place?

A. threefold

B. fourfold

C. fivefold

D. sixfold

E. no increased risk of recurrent symptoms.

D Studies show that patients who undergo semidefinitive
procedures that preserve the uninvolved ovary have a sixfold increase in the rate of symptom recurrence compared
to those who undergo a definitive total abdominal hysterectomy and bilateral salpingo-oophorectomy. These patients also have an eightfold reoperation rate to remove
the remaining ovary if it develops recurrent disease.

5. Why is it thought that women with endometriosis have
implantation defects?

A. They have a decreased expression of a specific integrin
produced during cycle days 20 to 24.

B. The endometrium is not in phase.

C. They have an increased risk for Asherman's syndrome.

D. Endometrial inflammation is present.

E. They have tubal distortion, which does not allow the zygote
to travel down the fallopian tube in the correct time frame.

A Specific integrins are known to express during the implantation window in the normal menstrual cycle, namely
days 20 to 24. One specific integrin, $\alpha v \beta 3$, has been
shown to be decreased in the endometrium of infertile
women with endometriosis, even though their endometrium is determined to be in phase by endometrial
biopsy. No findings of endometrial inflammation are
known, and women with endometriosis do not have a
higher risk for Asherman's syndrome. Patients with
endometriosis may have tubal distortion, but the role that
endometriosis may play in infertility is unclear, and many

patients have infertility with stage I or II endometriosis and do not have many pelvic adhesions. The general consensus is that the infertility/subfertility of these patients occurs on a more molecular level.

35

Evaluation of Amenorrhea

Kristy Ruis and Jeremy King

1. A 35-year-old woman presents with a 1-year history of amenorrhea. She reports that she delivered her third child over 8 months ago, is not lactating, and has not had a menstrual cycle. Upon further questioning, she states that she had rather significant bleeding after delivery, requiring curettage of the uterus. Each of the following could help confirm the diagnosis, *except:*

   A. LH
   B. FSH
   C. Growth hormone
   D. CBC

   > **D** Sheehan's syndrome, a cause of hypothalamic amenorrhea, is a condition of pituitary necrosis and hypopituitarism following postpartum hemorrhage and ensuing hypotension. Most commonly, deficiencies are seen in gonadotropins and growth hormone. Patients will experience amenorrhea, failure to lactate, and loss of pubic and axillary hair.

2. Patients with Turner syndrome will most commonly display which of the following endocrine profiles?

   A. Elevated TSH, normal FSH, normal prolactin
   B. Elevated FSH, normal TSH, normal prolactin
   C. Elevated prolactin, normal TSH, normal FSH
   D. Normal FSH, normal TSH, normal prolactin

B The majority of amenorrheic patients have a normal prolactin and TSH concentration. These women can be divided into those with an elevated FSH (gonadal failure) and those with a decreased or normal FSH (central origin or chronic anovulation). Gonadal dysgenesis is the most common cause of primary amenorrhea, accounting for 43% of such cases. Turner syndrome (TS), the most frequent cause of gonadal dysgenesis, is a condition in which all or part of one of the X chromosomes is missing. Sixty percent of TS patients are 45,X. The other 40% include various chromatin-positive karyotypes, most commonly 45,X/46,XX and 46,XXqi. Normal development of internal and external female genitalia occurs in utero. However, the cohort of primordial follicles undergoes accelerated atresia so that oocytes are depleted long before the onset of puberty. In the majority of TS patients, a lack of gonadal estrogen production results in a failure of secondary sexual development.

3. A patient presents with primary amenorrhea. She is found to have low levels of circulating FSH, LH, and estrogen. She has a normal female karyotype and negligible sexual development. Which of the following might also be noted in this patient?

   A. Loss of visual acuity

   B. Loss of auditory sense

   C. Anosmia

   D. Lack of proprioception

   C Kallmann syndrome, a form of hypothalamic amenorrhea, is an inherited disorder resulting from a genetic mutation that causes failure of olfactory and GnRH neuronal migration from the olfactory placode. Kallmann's syndrome is characterized by primary amenorrhea, a normal female karyotype with negligible sexual development, and anosmia. The absence of pulsatile secretions of GnRH results in low levels of FSH, LH, and low estrogen levels.

4. A 15-year-old patient with a diagnosis of Mayer-Rokitansky-Küster-Hauser (MRKH) syndrome is referred to you because of cyclic pelvic pain. You may counsel the patient that

   A. The pain cannot be real because she does not have any pelvic structures.

B. She does not require any imaging of the urinary tract.

C. Skeletal abnormalities are uncommon with this disorder.

D. Her pain may be related to the presence of a rudimentary müllerian structure with functioning endometrium.

D Müllerian agenesis, also known as Mayer-Rokitansky-Küster-Hauser (MRKH) syndrome, is the second most common cause of primary amenorrhea. The incidence is 1:5,000. Subjects with MRKH commonly present in their later teens with normal secondary sexual development. Amenorrhea is generally the only complaint, although 2% to 7% may have rudimentary müllerian structures with functioning endometrium resulting in cyclic pain. As mentioned previously, determining whether a uterus is present in a subject with breast development and primary amenorrhea is essential. Imaging of the urinary tract should be performed in all patients with vaginal agenesis, because approximately 30% have renal anomalies. Skeletal abnormalities are also commonly associated with MRKH.

5. Which of the following statements about amenorrhea is most correct?

A. The majority of amenorrheic patients have an abnormal physical exam, prolactin, or TSH concentration.

B. Imperforate hymen is the second most common cause of primary amenorrhea.

C. Gonadal dysgenesis is the most common cause of primary amenorrhea.

D. The term *hypothalamic amenorrhea* applies to conditions in which GnRH secretion is normal but circulating gonadotropin levels are elevated.

C The majority of amenorrheic patients have a *normal* physical exam, prolactin, and TSH concentration. Gonadal dysgenesis is the most common cause of primary amenorrhea, accounting for 43% of such cases. Müllerian agenesis, or MRKH syndrome, is the second most common cause of primary amenorrhea. The term *hypothalamic amenorrhea* applies to conditions in which GnRH secretion is *diminished* (resulting in low circulating gonadotropin levels) in the absence of any organic pathology.

36

Abnormal Uterine Bleeding

Linda M. Szymanski and Kimberly B. Fortner

1. A 58-year-old, healthy, gravida 0 comes to your office complaining about her vaginal bleeding. On further inquiry, she reports hot flushes and mood swings starting about 10 years ago. She stopped bleeding a few years ago and then started having irregular "periods" approximately 6 months ago. The most likely diagnosis is

A. Endometrial polyps

B. Endometrial hyperplasia

C. Endometrial cancer

D. Endometrial atrophy

> **D** The patient described in this case is having postmenopausal bleeding. Though she describes the vaginal bleeding as "periods," her symptoms indicate that she started with perimenopausal symptoms 10 years ago and likely entered menopause shortly thereafter.
>
> The most common cause of all postmenopausal bleeding is endometrial atrophy (56%), leaving 15% with some form of hyperplasia and 7% to 10% with endometrial cancer (1,2). The patient is a gravida 0, which puts her at increased risk for hyperplasia or even cancer, but in the general healthy population, atrophy will still be the most likely diagnosis. Of course, the patient should undergo evaluation for the bleeding to rule out hyperplasia, cancers, polyps, or iatrogenic causes.

2. Imaging of a stable 38-year-old, gravida 2, para 2, with post-menstrual spotting, is *best* performed by which of the following tests?

    A. Transvaginal ultrasound alone, because this is a better diagnostic tool in premenopausal as compared to postmenopausal women

    B. Saline infusion sonography because it is the most sensitive noninvasive method for diagnosing polyps

    C. CT scanning of the pelvis due to its ability to diagnose premenopausal bleeding etiologies

    D. Hematology consult, given your high suspicion for coagulopathy

    B The stable reproductive-age woman with postmenstrual spotting is classically thought to have polyps. Saline infusion sonography is an excellent, noninvasive test to evaluate for both polyps and submucous fibroids. Its accuracy approaches that of office hysteroscopy (3), and it can be performed with minimal discomfort to the patient. Transvaginal sonography is a very useful tool to evaluate numerous etiologies. The statement in choice A is false because the transvaginal ultrasound is a better diagnostic tool in postmenopausal women than in premenopausal. CT scanning should be used when the suspicion for cancer is quite high to evaluate the abdomen and pelvis. A hematology consult is indicated when suspicion for coagulopathy is high. However, in an otherwise healthy 38-year-old woman with two children and no previous problems, a bleeding disorder is much less likely.

3. A consultation is requested for a 14-year-old with heavy vaginal bleeding in the Emergency Department. This is her first menstrual cycle and she reports that her bleeding has not stopped over the last 10 days. Other than a pregnancy test, the next most high yield test would be

    A. Thyroid stimulating hormone and free thyroxine

    B. Prolactin

    C. Ristocetin cofactor activity

    D. Follicle stimulating hormone (FSH)

    C Excessive bleeding with the first menses is very likely to represent a bleeding dyscrasia (4). In fact, coagulopathies should be suspected in a patient with menorrhagia refractory to conservative management with anemia, and in adolescent patients with bleeding heavy enough to require a blood transfusion. The bleeding problems that should be tested are not limited to von Willebrand's disease (vWD), but vWD is the most common inherited bleeding disorder. Tests for vWD include plasma VWF antigen, plasma VWF activity (ristocetin cofactor activity), activated partial thromboplastin time, factor VIII activity, and bleeding time. In women with vWD, menorrhagia is a typical manifestation of the disease and most often beginning at menarche.

Bleeding in an adolescent should always include evaluation for pregnancy. The most common cause for irregular menstrual bleeding in an adolescent is anovulation, resulting from an immature hypothalamic-pituitary-ovarian axis. If the diagnosis of dysfunctional uterine bleeding is considered in an adolescent, it would be appropriate to order FSH, LH, TSH, and prolactin on day 3 of the menstrual cycle.

4. A 43-year-old gravida 1 para 1 with morbid obesity, hypertension, and COPD comes to the office complaining of heavy vaginal bleeding. Workup reveals normal lab work, ultrasound, and endometrial biopsy. The patient desires the safest long-term management for her bleeding. The *best* option is

   A. Oral contraceptive pill (OCP) taper and then long-term OCP use

   B. NSAIDS because they may reduce menstrual volume by 80% to 90%

   C. Admission to the hospital for hysterectomy

   D. Discussion and placement of Mirena intrauterine device

   D Given her medical problems, the patient is not an ideal candidate for either estrogen or surgery, thus ruling out choices A and C. Choice B is incorrect in that NSAIDs may reduce volume of menstrual flow by 20% to 40% (5). A levonorgestrel releasing IUD is a safe option for this patient. The levonorgestrel releasing IUD has been shown to decrease menstrual blood loss by up to 90%. In this morbidly obese patient, a prudent action is to recognize her risk for development of future endometrial pathology (hyperplasia or cancer). Thus, the localized progesterone effect could offer even greater benefit (6).

References

1. Lidor A, Ismajovich B, Condino E, et al. Histopathologic findings in 226 women with postmenopausal uterine bleeding. *Acta Obstet Gynecol Scand* 1986;65:41–43.
2. Karlsson B, Granberg S, Wikland M, et al. Transvaginal ultrasonography of the endometrium in women with postmenopausal bleeding: a Nordic multicenter study. *Am J Obstet Gynecol* 1995; 172:1488–1494.
3. Kelekci S, Kaya E, Alan M, et al. Comparison of transvaginal sonography, saline infusion sonography, and office hysteroscopy in reproductive-aged women with or without abnormal uterine bleeding. *Fertil Steril* 2005;84:682–686.
4. Claessens EA, Cowell CA. Acute adolescent menorrhagia. *Am J Obstet Gynecol* 1981;139(3):277–280.
5. Lethaby A, Augood C, Duckitt K. Nonsteroidal anti-inflammatory drugs for heavy menstrual bleeding [*Cochrane Review*]. In The Cochrane Library, Issue 2, 2001.
6. Wildemeersch D, Dhont M. Treatment of nonatypical and atypical endometrial hyperplasia with a levonorgestrel-releasing intrauterine system. *Am J Obstet Gynecol* 2003;188(5):1297–1298.

37

Hyperandrogenism

Kimberly B. Fortner and Christopher W. Lipari

1. A 34-year-old woman presents complaining of increased body hair growth. She states that she has been noticing increased dark, fine hair on her arms and legs over the last 2 years. She has no other complaints and reports that none of her family has ever had increased hair growth. Her medical history is notable for seizure disorder, for which she takes Dilantin, hypertension, for which she takes lisinopril, and diabetes, for which she takes Glipizide. On exam, she has a normal breast and pelvic exam, and no hair appears on her face, chest, or back, only on her arms and legs. You

   A. Recommend chemical hair removal.

   B. Recommend a visit with her neurologist to discuss a change in her antiepileptic from Dilantin.

   C. Recommend a visit to her internist to change her antihypertensive to spironolactone, thus treating her hypertension and hair growth.

   D. Initiate finasteride and ask her to follow up in 3 months.

   E. Recommend that she accept the increased hair growth because it is part of the aging process.

   B The key to the proper treatment is identifying the type of increased hair growth. This woman has hypertrichosis, characterized by excessive growth of villus hair. This condition may be due to genetic factors or from exposure to medications (such as Dilantin). Cessation of the medication should help alleviate the increased hair growth.

   By her exam, clearly, the patient does not have hirsutism. Hirsutism refers to the growth of dark terminal hair on the face, chest, back, lower abdomen, and upper thighs caused by the overactivity of circulating androgen hormones. One possible treatment of hirsutism is spironolactone.

With age, some of the hair follicles in particular areas of the body produce thick, darkly pigmented hair in response to androgen exposure. This thick, dark hair is called *terminal hair*. The remaining hair follicles produce villus hair, which is finer than terminal hair and not as darkly pigmented. Hair follicles on the lower arms and legs do not respond to androgen stimulation and continue to produce villus hair.

Once increased hair growth has been properly evaluated, removal of the hair can be recommended.

2. A 46-year-old woman comes to your office worried about her decreased sexual desire and perimenopausal symptoms. Her medical and surgical history are significant only for right salpingo-oophorectomy 10 years ago. Upon performing her annual exam, you feel left adnexal fullness, and pelvic sonogram shows an 8-cm cyst. After discussion of potential removal of the ovary, the patient is very worried that removal of her remaining ovary will leave her with no testosterone. You tell her that

A. Nearly all testosterone production is from her remaining ovary and her concerns are justified.

B. One fourth of her testosterone production is from her ovary, one-fourth from her adrenals, and the remaining half from peripheral conversion.

C. Testosterone production is not linked to a woman's ovaries.

D. Given that she is perimenopausal, she likely has little testosterone circulating anyway.

B In women, nearly one fourth of testosterone is secreted from the ovaries and one fourth is from the adrenals. The remaining one half is produced from peripheral conversion of androstenedione, occurring in the kidney, liver, and adipose tissue.

Testosterone levels decrease by 50% from ages 20 to 40. During premenopausal years, production of testosterone decreases under the control of luteinizing hormone

(LH). As the menopausal period is entered, sex hormone binding globulin (SHBG) levels remain constant, yielding an even greater decrease in free testosterone. Throughout menopause no further decreases occur in testosterone, but levels of SHBG fall due to the lack of estrogen, finally resulting in an increase in bioavailable testosterone. This increase is such that testosterone levels in an 80-year-old woman are only 20% lower than those in a 20-year-old.

3. A 30-year-old woman presents reporting difficulty becoming pregnant. After your history, you discover that she has always had irregular menses that "regulated" with oral contraception, and review of systems reveals occasional palpitations that she attributes to anxiety attacks. On exam, she has slight increased hair growth on her face and is overweight, making evaluation of her adnexa difficult. In addition to pelvic ultrasound, appropriate laboratory evaluation could include all of the following, *except:*

   A. DHEAS and 17 hydroxyprogesterone
   B. Prolactin and thyroid-stimulating hormone
   C. Insulin function tests
   D. Testosterone and androstenedione
   E. Basic metabolic panel

   E The clinician should plan to check the following: Testosterone and androstenedione. It is now thought that free testosterone or the free testosterone index may be more sensitive due to the lack of normative data for androstenedione. DHEAS levels should also be done to assess adrenal gland androgen production. Levels >700 ng/dL are considered markers for abnormal adrenal function. 17α-hydroxyprogesterone (17-OHP) should be checked. Serum levels of 100 to 300 ng/dL are normal. Prolactin and thyroid function tests should be done to evaluate her amenorrhea and hot flushes. Normative serum levels for prolactin are 1 to 20 ng/mL. In thyroid function tests, elevated levels of prolactin or thyroid hormones may produce hyperandrogenism directly by affecting androgen production and indirectly by creating an anovulatory state. Consideration of insulin function tests should be given.

4. On ultrasound, the patient is found to have 14 small cysts on each ovary. Given her most likely diagnosis, the possible treatment to assist in her fertility would be:

A. Weight loss, possible use of metformin or clomiphene citrate.

B. Initiation of Synthroid

C. Initiation of spironolactone

D. Surgery to perform adnexectomy

A In 2003, the Rotterdam ESHRE/ASRM-sponsored PCOS consensus workshop revised the **diagnostic criteria** for PCOS to include two of the following three:

Oligomenorrhea and/or anovulation

Clinical and/or biochemical signs of hyperandrogenism

Polycystic ovaries and exclusion of other etiologies (HumRep vol 19, 2004).

Evidence of hyperandrogenism can be demonstrated either by hirsutism or measurement of elevated levels of androgens. Polycystic ovaries are defined as the presence of 12 or more follicles in each ovary measuring 2 to 9 mm and/or increased ovarian volume (>10 mL). Patients with hyperandrogenemic chronic anovulation syndrome present with hirsutism, oligomenorrhea, amenorrhea, obesity, infertility, and pelvic pain. All or only some of these symptoms may be present. **If pregnancy is desired** by individuals with hyperandrogenemic chronic anovulation syndrome, assistance with ovulation induction is frequently required. This assistance may be provided by the oral medication clomiphene citrate. Studies have shown that the use of the hypoglycemic agent metformin hydrochloride (500 mg three times daily), either alone or in combination with clomiphene citrate, may result in ovulation.

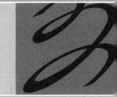

38

Female Sexual Function and Dysfunction

Scott C. Purinton and Andrew Goldstein

1. Treatment options for vulvar vestibulitis syndrome (VVS) include all of the following, *except:*

A. Lidocaine

B. Interferon

C. Vulvar vestibulectomy

D. Sildenafil

E. Capsaicin

> **D** Vulvar vestibulitis syndrome (VVS) is characterized by severe introital dyspareunia. The severe searing, knife-like pain that women feel with VVS is caused by a proliferation of C-afferent nociceptors in the vestibular mucosa. Treatments for VVS include topical lidocaine, capsaicin, nitroglycerine, intralesional interferon alpha, and oral tricyclic antidepressants (TCAs). If conservative treatments for VVS fail, excision of the vestibular tissue by the surgical procedure vulvar vestibulectomy, with vaginal advancement, is more than 80% effective if performed by a specialist in vulvar disease.

2. Treatment options for dysesthetic vulvodynia include all of the following, *except:*

A. Prozac

B. Venlafaxine

C. Biofeedback

D. Gabapentin

E. Botulinum toxin

B The symptoms of dysesthetic vulvodynia are caused by a combination of neuropathy, pelvic floor dysfunction, and central sensitization. Therefore, treatments for dysesthetic vulvodynia address these three components. Treatments for pelvic floor dysfunction include intravaginal physical therapy and biofeedback. In addition, recent studies have shown that intramuscular injections of botulinum toxin A (Botox) significantly improve pelvic floor hypertonicity. TCAs, such as amitriptyline and desipramine, or the selective serotonin and norepinephrine reuptake inhibitors (SSNRIs) duloxetine and venlafaxine, can be used to treat central sensitization. Anticonvulsants, such as gabapentin, topiramate, and carbamazepine, can be used to treat the neuropathic pain component of dysesthetic vulvodynia.

3. Illnesses that may cause female sexual dysfunction (FSD) may include all of the following, *except:*

A. Diabetes mellitus

B. Peripheral vascular disease

C. Multiple sclerosis

D. Sarcoidosis

E. Hyperprolactinemia

D The cause of FSD is almost always multifactorial and complex. The cause of a problem can be hormonal, vascular, neurologic, pharmacologic, or psychogenic, but the cause is more likely due to more than one factor. Estrogens, androgens, oxytocin, and dopaminergic agonists are believed to promote the female sexual response, whereas progesterone, prolactin, and serotonin play an inhibitory role. Hypertension, hypercholesterolemia, diabetes mellitus, and smoking all contribute to vascular injury of the small vessels of the vagina and clitoris.

4. Treatment options for hypoactive desire disorder include all of the following, *except:*

A. Bupropion

B. Testosterone cream

C. Estradiol

D. Oral contraceptive pills

E. Apomorphine

> **D** Oral contraceptive pills can actually have an inhibitory effect on female sexual function. Oral contraceptives pills (OCP) are the most prevalent form of birth control for women younger than age 35. Four randomized controlled studies have examined the effect of OCPs on sexual function. Three of these studies show a modest population-dependent decrease in sexual desire in OCP users. Also, the relatively high discontinuation rate of OCP use within the first 4 months after initiation may be partly due to decreased sexual function. OCPs increase serum levels of sex hormone-binding globulin, which binds to free serum testosterone and decreases the amount of circulating free testosterone. The decrease in testosterone leads to decreased sexual desire.

5. Treatment options for sexual arousal disorder include all of the following, *except:*

A. Eros CTD device

B. L-Arginine

C. Tadalafil

D. Intravaginal physical therapy

E. Prostaglandin E1

> **D** The treatments for sexual arousal disorder focus on increasing blood flow to the clitoris, vulva, and vagina. Intravaginal physical therapy, along with biofeedback, is used as a treatment for pelvic floor dysfunction, a component of dysesthetic vulvodynia.

39

Menopause and Hormone Replacement Therapy

Jennifer Kulp and Howard Zacur

1. A 50-year-old healthy woman presents to the office for a routine gynecologic visit. She complains of new onset of episodes of intense heat through her neck and chest followed by periods of profuse sweating. She is concerned because these episodes interfere with her ability to work and also wake her up from sleep. What is the most effective therapy for the symptoms the patient is describing?

   A. Venlafaxine
   B. Clonidine
   C. Estrogen replacement
   D. Black cohosh

   C The patient is most likely perimenopausal and is experiencing hot flashes. The average age of menopause is 50, with a range of 43 to 57 years. Seventy-five percent of menopausal women experience hot flashes. Vasomotor instability causes the hot flash, characterized by a sudden reddening of the skin over the head, neck, and chest, accompanied by a feeling of intense body heat, and concluding with profuse perspiration. Hot flashes may also cause sleep disturbances and irritability.

   Estrogen administration is the most effective treatment for hot flashes and is administered orally, transdermally, or vaginally. In women with a uterus, progestins must be added to any estrogen regimen to prevent the increased risk of endometrial cancer associated with unopposed estrogen use. Current recommendations state that estrogen should be used for the shortest duration possible for the relief of hot flashes. Women with a history of venous thromboembolism or stroke, or those at high risk for developing these conditions or women with a history of breast cancer or coronary heart disease, are not candidates for systemic estrogen therapy. For these women alternative therapies exist, such as the serotonin reuptake inhibitors venlafaxine and paroxetine. Clonidine may also be used to control hot flash symptoms in women who are not candidates for estrogen. Black cohosh, although approved in Europe for the treatment of hot flashes, needs more study to determine its usefulness and side effects in the treatment of hot flashes.

2. A 62-year-old woman presents to your office complaining of discomfort and pain with intercourse, which she notes has developed over the past few years. A physical exam reveals atrophic vaginal mucosa. What initial therapy would you recommend for this patient?

   A. A vaginal lubricant, such as Replens

   B. Transdermal estrogen

   C. Marriage counseling

   D. Oral hormone replacement therapy

   A Dyspareunia is the most common complaint related to vaginal atrophy. Moisturizers and lubricants, such as Replens, Astroglide, and K-Y jelly may be used to relieve symptoms related to vaginal dryness and dyspareunia. Astroglide and K-Y jelly are used at the time of coitus to alleviate dyspareunia, whereas Replens is used on a sustained basis. These lubricants may first be tried for vaginal atrophy secondary to estrogen deficiency. However, local estrogen therapy remains the mainstay of therapy for urogenital atrophy. Estrogen creams or tablets are applied intravaginally and estrogenize the vaginal mucosa. Transdermal or oral estrogen are not currently recommended for the treatment of urogenital atrophy.

3. A new patient comes to your office for a routine gynecologic visit. She is a 57-year-old African American woman who has been postmenopausal since age 50. She denies any medical problems but mentions that she fractured her hip 2 years ago. On exam, she is 5 feet, 5 inches tall and weighs 165 pounds. Physical findings are significant for slightly atrophic vaginal

mucosa but otherwise normal exam. In addition to doing a pap smear and ordering a mammogram, you give the patient a referral for a DEXA because of her

A. Race

B. Postmenopausal status combined with physical exam findings

C. History of a fracture

D. Height and weight

C Bone mineral density (BMD) should be measured in any postmenopausal patient who presents with a fracture. Other candidates for BMD determination are all women older than age 65. The U. S. Preventive Services Task Force recommends beginning screening at age 60 for women who have risk factors for osteoporosis. Although the patient is postmenopausal, she is only 57 years old, so that in itself would be a reason for screen. Low body weight, which is considered a weight under 70 kg (154 pounds), is not a risk factor for this patient.

4. A 50-year-old woman presents to your office complaining of hot flashes. Her friend tried hormone replacement therapy (HRT), which helped to relieve her hot flashes, and your patient wants more information. She states, "Didn't that study say that women shouldn't take hormones any more"? You tell her that the Women's Health Initiative (WHI) study showed that

A. Women on HRT have a decreased amount of hot flashes.

B. Women on HRT have a decreased risk of cognitive decline.

C. Women on HRT have no significant decreased risk of osteoporosis related fractures compared to placebo.

D. Women on HRT have an increased risk of stroke.

D The WHI study was designed to look at a primary outcome of the risk of heart disease. It enrolled women older than age 59. Women with menopausal symptoms, such as hot flashes, were discouraged from participating in the study, and the effect of HRT on hot flashes was not evaluated. Initial results reported an increased risk of heart disease among hormone users. However, a follow-up study that reviewed all cardiovascular events found no statistical difference in cardiovascular events between placebo and hormone users. An increased risk of stroke, of approximately 0.5% to 1.0%, in women on HRT, was demonstrated. This study demonstrated a reduction in hip and vertebral fractures in women on HRT compared to placebo. The WHI points out that HRT does not decrease the risk of cognitive decline in postmenopausal women. However, HRT remains the most effective treatment for menopausal signs and symptoms. Current recommendations state that estrogen should be used for the shortest duration possible for the relief of hot flashes.

40

Diseases of the Vulva

Julie Phillips, Kamal Hamod, and Robert L. Giuntoli, II

1. A 28-year-old P0 presents to your office for her annual exam. She has no complaints. On examination, you note a 1-cm soft fluctuant nodule on the medial aspect of her left labia minora at the 5 o'clock position of the hymenal ring. It is nonerythematous and nontender to palpation. Which of the following treatment options would you advise?

A. Sitz baths and antibiotics

B. Insertion of a Word catheter

C. Marsupialization

D. Do nothing

> **D** This patient has a Bartholin's gland cyst. These cysts are relatively common and require no treatment if uninfected and the patient is asymptomatic. Bartholin's gland cysts can become infected. Infections are usually polymicrobial but 10% are caused by Neisseria gonorrhea. Drainage is necessary for abscesses. Word catheter placement is more effective than simple incision and drainage. Recurrent abscess formation may require gland marsupialization.

2. A 25-year-old woman presents to your office complaining of thick, white, vaginal discharge as well as vulvar itching and burning. Her past medical history is significant for diabetes mellitus and asthma, and she recently finished a course of amoxicillin for an ear infection. She is sexually active and uses

oral contraceptive pills. Which of the following is not a risk factor for her symptoms?

A. Diabetes

B. Recent use of antibiotics

C. Sexual activity

D. Use of oral contraceptives

> **C** This patient has a yeast infection, most commonly caused by candida albicans. Candida infections are not considered to be sexually transmitted; therefore sexual activity does not increase the risk of developing a yeast infection. Diabetes, recent use of broad-spectrum antibiotics, and use of oral contraceptives all increase the risk of developing a yeast infection. Other risk factors are immunosuppression, pregnancy, and use of steroids.

3. A 75-year-old woman presents to your office complaining of vulvar pruritus. On examination you note a 2-cm hypopigmented lesion on the posterior fourchette. What is the most appropriate next step in management?

A. Vulvar biopsy

B. Hydrocortisone cream

C. Estrogen cream

D. Do nothing

> **A** It is difficult to differentiate benign from malignant vulvar lesions, especially in the elderly. Any suspicious lesion should be first biopsied to rule out vulvar cancer. Punch biopsies can be performed easily in the office. Only if the lesion is identified as benign can symptomatic treatment with estrogen or hydrocortisone cream be initiated.

4. A 69-year-old woman with a recent diagnosis of vulvar cancer is referred to your office to discuss treatment options. She asks if she will be receiving radiation therapy. You tell her that radiation therapy may be useful but that it depends on the type of cancer she has. In which type of vulvar carcinoma is radiation therapy contraindicated?

A. Basal cell carcinoma

B. Verrucous carcinoma

C. Melanoma

D. Paget's disease of the vulva

> **B** Verrucous carcinoma is a variant of squamous carcinoma of the vulva. It presents as a large fungating mass and local destruction is common. Treatment requires radical local excision. Radiation therapy is contraindicated as it may induce increased aggression in malignant activity. Wide local excision is used to treat basal cell carcinoma, melanoma, and Paget's disease. However, radiation therapy can be used in aggressive disease.

5. A 48-year-old P2002 is referred to your clinic after seeing multiple physicians for vulvar pain and burning. She has been unable to have intercourse or wear tampons for the past year because the pain is so severe. She has been treated with multiple courses of antibiotics and antifungal medications without relief. Her most likely diagnosis is

A. Urinary tract infection

B. Vulvar neuropathy

C. Vulvar vestibulitis syndrome

D. Levator ani myalgia

> **C** This woman is most likely experiencing vulvar vestibulitis syndrome, a chronic inflammation of the vestibular glands characterized by severe pain elicited by touch. A urinary tract infection would be characterized by dysuria, urinary urgency, and frequency. Vulvar neuropathy is constant burning pain, not only elicited by touch. Finally, levator ani myalgia is characterized by spasm of the pelvic floor muscles, usually manifesting itself after minor trauma to the area.

41

Cervical Intraepithelial Neoplasia

Colleen McCormick

1. Which patients require a repeat pap in 6 months if their pap returns without evidence of intraepithelial lesion but with no endocervical cells present?

A. HIV+

B. History of LSIL pap 6 years ago with normal paps since

C. Last pap was ASCUS

D. A and B

E. A and C

E If the pap smear is inadequate by virtue of having no endocervical cells but no risk factors are present, repeat pap smear can be deferred for a year. However, if any risk factors are present, a pap smear should be repeated in 6 months. Risk factors include a history ASCUS or greater abnormalities in the past without three interval normal pap smears, a history of positive HPV cytology within the last 6 months, a history of a glandular abnormality, an immunocompromised state, inability to visualize the endocervical canal, and a noncompliant patient.

2. Which patient does not require colposcopy?

A. Pap ASCUS, HPV+

B. Pap ASCUS, HPV−

C. History of LSIL with colposcopy CIN1/adequate 12 months ago, now again with pap LSIL

D. AGC pap

E. HSIL pap

B The three strategies for managing ASCUS pap smears are HPV testing, reflex colposcopy, and repeat pap smear. If reflex testing for high risk HPV is used, HPV+ should be considered equivalent to LSIL, and the patient should be referred to colposcopy. One million women a year in the United States will have CIN1. Spontaneous regression occurs in 57% of immunocompetent patients, 30% will persist, 11% will progress to CIN2/3, and 0.3% will progress to cervical cancer. Therefore, these lesions can be followed conservatively once colposcopy has been performed and CIN1 is confirmed. Follow-up options include repeating a pap smear at 6 and 12 months, with repeat colposcopy for ASCUS or greater. This approach detects 85% of CIN3, and 60% of women will require a further colposcopy. Another option is HPV testing at 12 months, with repeat colposcopy if high risk types are present. This option detects 95% of CIN3, and 55% of women will require another colposcopy. Another recommended triage option is repeat colposcopy and pap smear at 12 months. All women with AGC on pap smear should be referred to colposcopy and an endocervical curetting (ECC) should be performed. A woman with an HSIL pap smear will have CIN2/3 70% to 75% of the time and an invasive cancer 1% to 2% of the time. All HSIL pap smears should trigger colposcopy with ECC.

3. An excisional procedure is not recommended in which of the following patients?

   A. AGC favor neoplasia with negative colposcopy and endometrial biopsy

   B. 16 year old with LSIL on two paps, colposcopy CIN1, adequate

   C. HSIL on pap, CIN2, inadequate colposcopy

   D. LSIL pap, inadequate colposcopy

   B AGC favor neoplasia carries a relatively high risk of invasive disease. Although a glandular abnormality is possible, CIN is the most frequent diagnosis after an AGC pap smear. However, of AGC pap smears, 0% to 8% will have adenocarcinoma in situ on biopsy, and 1% to 9% will have invasive cancer. All women with AGC on pap smear should be referred to colposcopy and an endocervical curetting (ECC) should be performed. If the woman is over age 35 or has abnormal bleeding, an endometrial biopsy should also be performed. If the pap smear was AGC-favor neoplasia and no abnormalities are found with this preliminary workup, a cold knife cone (CKC) should be performed. If the initial pap smear was AGC-NOS and initial workup is negative, pap smears should be repeated every 4 to 6 months until four are normal, and then routine screening can be resumed. If AGC is persistent, a CKC should be performed. While in immunocompetent women, untreated CIN2 will regress 43% of the time, 35% will persist, and 22% will progress to invasive cancer. Therefore, these lesions should be treated, and, for treatment to be effective, the whole transformation zone should be excised. Patients with a satisfactory colposcopy and CIN2/3 can be treated with either an excisional procedure or an ablative one, although excision is usually preferred to rule out microinvasion. Ablation should only be done if no discrepancy exists between the cytology, colposcopy, or histology; if the lesion is limited to the endocervix and is seen in its entirety; and if no evidence of endocervical involvement on ECC is present. Cancer is found in 0.5% of excisional specimens done for CIN2/3, with a satisfactory colposcopy. Up to 7% of patients with CIN2/3 and unsatisfactory colposcopy will be found to have a microinvasive lesion. Therefore, all such cases should be treated with an excisional procedure. All CIN1 lesions with unsatisfactory colposcopy require a diagnostic excisional procedure. (Although, in the face of an otherwise reassuring colposcopy and a compliant patient, some practitioners would follow conservatively with serial colposcopy and pap smears.) For CIN1 confirmed by adequate colposcopy, the risk of progression to invasive disease is low and the rate of regression is high: Spontaneous regression occurs in 57% of immunocompetent patients, 30% will persist, 11% will progress to CIN2/3, and 0.3% will progress to cervical cancer. These lesions can therefore be followed conservatively. This scenario is especially true in younger patients in whom the rate of HPV infection is high, but the rate of invasive cancer is low.

42

Cervical Cancer

Katherine Goodrich and Teresa P. Díaz-Montes

1. Cervical cancer is staged

  A. Clinically

  B. Surgically

  C. Clinically and surgically

  D. None of the above

> **A** Cervical cancer is staged clinically. Staging of cervical cancer is based on clinical, rather than surgical, evaluation. The following examinations are permitted: inspection, palpation, colposcopy, endocervical curettage (ECC), hysteroscopy, cystoscopy, proctoscopy, intravenous urography, and radiographic examination of the chest and skeleton. Biopsies of the cervix, bladder, or rectum should be performed for histologic evidence. Conization or amputation of the cervix is considered a clinical examination in the setting of cervical cancer staging. Inspection, palpation, and studies, such as colposcopy, ECC, hysteroscopy, cystoscopy, and sigmoidoscopy, should be performed by an experienced examiner, preferably while the patient is under anesthesia. Because the most common sites of distant spread include the lungs and skeleton, radiographic examination of the chest and skeleton is warranted. Patients with hydronephrosis or nonfunctioning kidneys demonstrated by imaging studies are automatically assigned to stage IIIB.

2. Clinical trials have demonstrated that the best radiosensitizing agent in cervical cancer treatment is

  A. 5-FU

B. Bleomycin
C. Taxol
D. Cisplatin
E. Vincristine

> **D** Clinical trials have demonstrated that the best radiosensitizing agent in cervical cancer treatment is cisplatin. The use of chemoradiation has become widely recognized as providing survival benefit over radiation alone in the treatment of cervical cancer, based on the theory of synergistic cell kill. When combined with radiation, weekly cisplatin administration reduces the risk of progression for stage IIB through stage IVA cervical cancer. Similarly, in patients with bulky IB disease treated with concurrent cisplatin/radiation versus radiation alone and hysterectomy at the completion of radiation, disease recurrence over 36 months of follow-up was 21% in the group treated with concurrent chemoradiation and 37% in the radiation alone group.

3. Pregnant patients with microinvasive cervical cancer may deliver vaginally. Is this statement true or false?

> **TRUE** Pregnant patients with microinvasive cervical cancer may deliver vaginally. In patients with carcinoma in situ or microinvasive disease stages IA1 or IA2, there appears to be no harm in delaying definitive therapy until after fetal maturity has been attained. Patients with less than 3 mm of invasion and no lymph vascular space involvement may be followed to term and delivered vaginally. The major risk to the patient during delivery through a cervix containing invasive carcinoma is the risk of hemorrhage due to tearing of the tumor during cervical dilation and delivery. Recurrences of cervical cancer have been reported at the episiotomy site in women who deliver vaginally. Following vaginal delivery, these women should be re-evaluated and treated at 6 weeks postpartum.

4. The most important factor in prognosis of cervical cancer is

A. Histologic type
B. Lymph vascular space involvement
C. Tumor grade
D. Stage
E. Age at diagnosis

D Although several prognostic variables exist, including age, race, socioeconomic status, immune status, and tumor characteristics, the most important factor is clinical stage. Conflicting data are known on the influence of histologic subtype on prognosis, and the relationship between lymph vascular space involvement and survival is not clear. When compared to well-differentiated tumors, those that are poorly differentiated have lower 5-year survival rates.

5. Risk factors for cervical cancer include

   A. Age at first intercourse

   B. Use of tobacco or exposure to second-hand smoke

   C. Infection with HPV

   D. Infection with *Chlamydia*

   E. Immunosuppression

   F. Race

   G. Socioeconomic status

   H. None of the above

   I. All of the above

I All choices are correct. First intercourse before age 16 is associated with a twofold increase in risk of cervical cancer compared with women with first intercourse after the age 20.

Cigarette smoking has been found to be an independent risk factor in the development of cervical disease, with smokers having a 4.5-fold increased risk of carcinoma in situ (CIS) compared with matched controls. Smokers also have a twofold to fourfold increased risk of cervical intraepithelial neoplasia type 3 (CIN 3) and invasive cervical cancer in women who were also infected with oncogenic HPV. Infection with specific high-risk papilloma virus (HPV) is the most important risk factor for the development of cervical cancer. Multiple studies have demonstrated that infection with *Chlamydia trachomatis* also increases the risk of developing invasive squamous cell carcinoma of the cervix. Immunocompromised women may be at higher risk of developing the disease and may demonstrate more rapid progression from preinvasion to invasive lesions. Patients who test positive for human immunodeficiency virus infection (HIV) appear to present with invasive cervical cancer earlier than patients who test negative for the virus and with more advanced disease at the time of diagnosis when CD4 cell counts are reduced (below 200/mm^3).

The incidence rate of cervical cancer among African Americans in the United States is higher than that among white women, with approximately 11 new cases per 100,000 blacks and 8 cases per 100,000 whites per year. The incidence is even higher in the Hispanic population, with approximately 14 new cases per 100,000 each year. Native Americans are estimated to have incidence rates similar to Hispanics. Asian groups experience rates similar to or lower than those of whites. A strong inverse association is found between cervical cancer incidence and socioeconomic factors. When socioeconomic differences are controlled for, the excess risk of cervical cancer among African Americans decreases.

43

Cancer of the Uterine Corpus

Colleen McCormick

1. Which of the following is not a risk factor for endometrial cancer?

A. Hereditary nonpolyposis cancer (HNPCC)

B. Obesity

C. Tamoxifen use

D. Birth control pill use

E. Nulliparity

D A woman's risk of endometrial cancer increases with age. Other risk factors are based on increased estrogen. Estrogen replacement without concomitant progesterone carries a relative risk of 4.5% to 8.0% and persists for 10 years after treatment is stopped. Chronic anovulation, such as seen in polycystic ovarian syndrome (PCOS), leads to constant estrogen stimulation of the endometrium and increases the risk of cancer. Obesity is felt to increase endogenous estrogen by increasing the peripheral levels of androstenedione that is then converted to estrogen by aromatase in adipose tissues. A woman taking tamoxifen has an annual risk of 2/1,000 of developing endometrial cancer. Women with hereditary nonpolyposis cancer (HNPCC) syndrome have up to a 50% lifetime risk of developing endometrial cancer. Factors that decrease circulating estrogen, such as cigarette smoking and OCP use, decrease this risk. OCPs decrease risk by 40% even up to 15 years after discontinuation, and this protection increases with length of use. Four years of use reduces risk by 56%, 8 years decreases risk by 67%, and 12 years decreases risk by 72%.

2. In a 65-year-old woman with postmenopausal bleeding, the most likely cause is

A. Endometrial cancer

B. Atrophy

C. Hyperplasia

D. Cervical source

> **B** Endometrial cancer often presents as postmenopausal bleeding, and all postmenopausal bleeding should be investigated. However, most postmenopausal bleeding is not caused by cancer. In one study of women with postmenopausal bleeding, 7% had cancer, 56% had atrophy, and 15% had endometrial hyperplasia. The likelihood that postmenopausal bleeding is due to cancer significantly increases with a woman's age. One study showed that 9% of women in their 50s, with postmenopausal bleeding, had endometrial cancer, whereas the rate was 16% for women in their 60s, 28% for women in their 70s, and 60% for women in their 80s.

3. If uterine papillary serous carcinoma is suspected on the frozen section, which additional procedure(s) should be performed?

A. Omentectomy

B. Pelvic and periaortic lymph node dissection

C. Appendectomy

D. Cholecystectomy

E. A and B

F. A and C

> **E** The presence of invasion to the outer one-third of the myometrium, high grade, clear cell histology, papillary serous histology, tumor greater than 2 cm in size, lymphvascular space invasion, cervical or lower uterine segment invasion, clinically bulky lymph nodes, or disease outside of the uterus should prompt lymph node dissection if deemed surgically possible. With the presence of any of these risk factors, the risk of positive lymph nodes increases to greater than 10%, and 5-year survival decreases to 70% to 85% without further treatment. Uterine papillary serous (UPSC) tends to metastasize early (72% have extrauterine spread at the time of diagnosis)

and metastasize more like an ovarian cancer. Therefore, omentectomy should be performed as part of surgical staging for a known UPSC. Although an appendectomy may be clinically appropriate, if the appendix is involved, this procedure is not required for complete staging or treatment.

4. Which of the following intraoperative findings should prompt lymph node dissection?

A. Invasion to 6 out of 11 mm, endometrioid type FIGO grade 1

B. UPSC, 2/10 mm invasion

C. FIGO grade 1, endocervical involvement

D. 4 cm tumor in the fundus, grade 1 with lymphvascular space invasion

E. All of the above

E The decision as to whether to proceed to lymph node dissection is often made in the operating room based on frozen section. The presence of invasion to the outer one-third of the myometrium, high grade, clear cell histology, papillary serous histology, tumor greater than 2 cm in size, lymphvascular space invasion, cervical or lower uterine segment invasion, clinically bulky lymph nodes, or disease outside of the uterus should prompt lymph node dissection if deemed surgically possible. Women without any of these risk factors have a less than 10% risk of positive lymph nodes and greater than 90% 5-year survival rate with just a TAH-BSO. However, with the presence of any of these risk factors, the risk of positive lymph nodes increases to greater than 10%, and 5-year survival decreases to 70% to 85% without further treatment.

44

Ovarian Cancer

Joel Larma and Ginger J. Gardner

1. A 47-year-old G3 P3003 presents to your office with vague complaints, including lower abdominal cramping, fullness, and a sensation that her abdominal girth has increased over the last several months. A comprehensive history reveals that the patient is menopausal but is otherwise healthy. She reports having had three uncomplicated vaginal deliveries and a postpartum tubal ligation with her last child. Her family history is significant only for a maternal aunt with breast cancer. The patient did give a history of using oral contraceptive pills (OCPs) for approximately 10 years before the birth of her first child. In this particular patient, all of the following are protective against ovarian cancer, *except*:

A. Multiparity

B. Breast-feeding

C. Family history of breast cancer

D. Bilateral tubal ligation

E. Oral contraceptive use

C Several protective factors exist against ovarian cancer. Multiparity reduces the risk of ovarian cancer, whereas a history of nulliparity and infertility increase the risk. Breast-feeding also appears protective. Over the years, OCPs have demonstrated several benefits aside from fertility control. The use of OCPs has been shown to dramatically reduce the risk of ovarian cancer and has been recommended in certain high risk populations, such as those women with a BRCA1 or BRCA 2 mutation. Along with a history of hysterectomy, bilateral tubal ligation appears protective against the development of ovarian cancer. Of the following answers, only a family history of breast cancer is not protective. A history of breast cancer in the family may be indicative of a hereditary form of ovarian cancer, including a mutation in one of the BRCA genes or hereditary nonpolyposis cancer syndrome.

2. A careful physical examination reveals a protuberant abdomen with moderate distention. On bimanual examination, a palpable left adnexal mass is present and rectovaginal examination is confirmatory. The patient is sent for blood work and imaging. The blood work was notable for an elevated CA-125 level at 155 U/mL.

CA-125 may be elevated in all of the following conditions, *except*:

A. Pelvic inflammatory disease

B. Endometriosis

C. Pregnancy

D. Hemorrhagic ovarian cysts

E. Pelvic organ prolapse (POP)

> **E** The clinical use of CA-125 as a screening tool for ovarian cancer has been hampered by its elevation in conditions other than ovarian cancer. Many gynecologic conditions are associated with an elevated CA-125 level, including pelvic inflammatory disease, endometriosis, pregnancy, and hemorrhagic ovarian cysts. Pelvic organ prolapse has not been associated with an elevated CA-125 level. Although CA-125 is not useful as a screening test for ovarian cancer, it is often used to monitor the efficacy of chemotherapy.

3. The patient undergoes an exploratory laparotomy, total abdominal hysterectomy, bilateral salpingo-oophorectomy and complete surgical staging. The surgical debulking was considered optimal. The final pathology reveals a well- differentiated, grade 1, stage IA, clear cell, ovarian carcinoma.

Which of the following portends a poor prognosis for this patient?

A. Optimal debulking

B. Surgical stage

C. Tumor histology

D. Age of patient

C Several variables affect prognosis in patients with epithelial ovarian cancer. In this patient, the final pathology revealed a well-differentiated, grade 1 tumor. Survival rates are higher in patients with lower grade tumors. Patients who are considered to have an optimal surgical debulking are those in whom the largest diameter of residual tumor is less than 1 cm. Patients have longer 5-year survival rates when their tumor is optimally debulked. As with most gynecologic malignancies, the prognosis varies based on the stage of the tumor with lower stages affording better outcomes. Furthermore, younger patients have higher survival rates than older patients. Of the various histologic types of epithelial ovarian carcinoma, only clear cell carcinoma is associated with poor prognosis.

4. The patient presents several years later to the clinic with complaints of progressively worsening nausea, bilious vomiting, and failure to pass flatus or stool. Examination reveals a moderately distended abdomen that is tympanic to percussion. Abdominal roentgenogram reveals dilated loops of bowel with numerous air-fluid levels. Vital signs and laboratory values are within normal limits.

Which of the following would be the appropriate next step in management?

A. Abdominal radiation therapy

B. Intravenous fluids with nasogastric tube decompression

C. Emergent exploratory laparotomy

D. Cisplatin-based chemotherapy

E. Outpatient follow-up

B A potential complication of ovarian carcinoma is bowel obstruction. The obstruction can be related to either a mechanical blockage or from carcinomatous ileus. The initial management of a small bowel obstruction should be conservative, using IVF, bowel rest, and possibly nasogastric decompression. Repletion of any electrolyte abnormalities should also be performed. With failure of conservative management, the patient may be a candidate for surgical exploration. If the patient is unlikely to benefit from a lengthy surgical resection or bypass, palliative care with possible gastrostomy tube placement can be used.

5. Several years later the patient's 20-year-old nulliparous daughter presents with complaints of chronic abdominal and pelvic pain. An ultrasound reveals a complex right adnexal mass. An exploratory laparotomy and a right salpingo-oophorectomy are performed. The frozen section reveals a well-differentiated dysgerminoma. The contralateral ovary is examined, and an excisional biopsy is negative for tumor. Full staging is performed, and all biopsies are negative for tumor.

Which of the following would be the appropriate next step in management?

A. BEP (Bleomycin, etoposide, and cisplatin) $\times$ 4 to 6 cycles

B. Palliative care

C. Tandem and ovoid radiation

D. Pelvic exenteration

E. Close follow-up, with physical exams and imaging

E Dysgerminomas are the most common ovarian germ cell tumors. They are frequently found in premenopausal women, particularly in the second decade of life. Treatment involves either a salpingo-oophorectomy or TAH/BSO. The former is generally performed when fertility is an issue, whereas the latter is reserved for those individuals in whom childbearing is complete. Pelvic exenteration is not generally performed, particularly when fertility is an issue. Dysgerminomas are particularly responsive to radiation therapy, but fertility is often compromised. These tumors are also sensitive to platinum-based chemotherapy but it is usually reserved for disease greater than stage IA. Tandem and ovoid radiation therapy is not helpful for management of dysgerminomas and is generally used for patients with cervical cancer.

Gestational Trophoblastic Disease

Ruchi Garg and Robert L. Giuntoli, II

1. The family of a 42-year-old P0020 Asian woman brings her to the emergency room with altered mental status. Upon further history taking, she is noted as having been diagnosed with a molar pregnancy about 6 months ago, for which she had undergone dilation and curettage. Patient's history is also notable for two previous spontaneous abortions, otherwise unremarkable. Workup reveals blood type O+, hemoglobin level of 9, β-HCG of 200,000.

All of the following are associated risk factors for a gestational trophoblastic disease for this patient, *except:*

A. Asian origin

B. Age over 40

C. History of spontaneous abortions

D. Blood type O+

D An increased risk of a hydatidiform mole is present at both extremes of reproductive age. Women older than age 40 have a 5.2-fold increased risk. An obstetric history of spontaneous abortion is more common in patients with GTD than in women without such a history. Asian race is also a risk factor and is associated with an increased risk of 1.8- to 2.1-fold. An association has been reported between ABO blood group and choriocarcinoma (but not hydatidiform mole), with blood group A being the most prevalent and blood group O as the least prevalent.

Head CT with contrast reveals an enhancement on the frontal lobe. After ruling out other possibilities, patient is presumed to have persistent gestational trophoblastic disease, that is, choriocarcinoma with metastasis.

2. Early systemic hematogenous metastasis with choriocarcinoma has been noted in all of the following organs, *except:*

A. Spine

B. Lungs

C. Liver

D. Brain

> **A** Eighty percent of the patients with metastatic disease show pulmonary involvement. Approximately, 30% of patients with extrauterine disease experience vaginal involvement; 10% of the patients with metastatic disease have the involvement of the liver. CNS disease is also seen in 10% of patients, mostly in those with advanced disease. These CNS lesions may undergo spontaneous hemorrhage, leading to acute focal neurologic deficits.
>
> Further workup revealed diffusely metastatic disease.

3. The recommended treatment that should be offered to the patient in questions 1 and 2 is:

A. Single agent chemotherapy with methotrexate

B. Chemotherapy regimen EMA-CO, along with whole-brain irradiation

C. Whole brain irradiation only

D. Hysterectomy

> **B** For patients with high-risk metastatic disease, the recommended treatment is combination chemotherapy with etoposide, methotrexate, actinomycin D, cyclophosphamide (Cytoxan), and vincristine sulfate (EMA-CO). For patients with complications of metastatic disease, including brain, whole-brain irradiation (approximately 3,000 cGy) is initiated as soon as the extent of disease is confirmed. Radiation and chemotherapy reduce the risk of spontaneous cerebral hemorrhage. Craniotomy is infrequently performed for acute decompression or acute bleeding in cases in which there is hope of survival and cure is probable.

4. A 21-year-old woman comes in for her first prenatal visit. Her last menstrual period was 12 weeks ago of which she is certain. Upon examination you note a 20-week uterus, therefore an ultrasound is performed and reveals bilaterally enlarged adnexa and a "snowstorm" pattern in the uterus. You order a serum β-HCG level, which comes back as 100,000, confirming your suspicion of a complete mole. Of course, the definite diagnosis will not be made until a D&C is performed. Clinical features that help distinguish a complete mole from a partial mole are

A. Gestational age between 8 and 16 weeks

B. B-HCG level of 100,000

C. Uterine size that is large for gestational age

D. Ultrasonographic features

E. All of the above

> **E** A complete mole is distinguished from a partial mole, based on several clinical features, including a classic "snowstorm" pattern on ultrasound with theca lutein cysts, large-for-gestational-age uterine size, β-HCG level >50K with gestational age between 8 and 16 weeks. Incomplete or partial mole rarely has the previously mentioned ultrasonographic features and is more commonly associated with a uterine size that is small for gestational age.

5. To optimally prepare for the D&C you should take the following steps, *except:*

A. Type and cross for blood

B. Full operating room setting

C. Suction cannula

D. General anesthesia

E. A 22-gauge intravenous access

> **E** The primary treatment for hydatidiform mole is suction D&C. Uterine evacuation is accomplished with the largest plastic cannula that can be safely introduced through the cervix. Arrangements should be made for a full operating room support in a hospital setting. Large-bore intravenous access should be initiated with ready access to typed and crossed blood products.

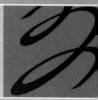

46

Chemotherapy and Radiation Therapy

Ruchi Garg and Edward Trimble

1. A 65-year-old woman is diagnosed with ovarian carcinoma. During surgical exploration, she is noted to have a 3-cm superficial liver lesion consistent with metastatic disease. Based on these findings, what stage of ovarian cancer should be assigned to the patient?

A. Stage IIIA

B. Stage IIIC

C. Stage IV

D. None of the above

B For ovarian cancer staging, superficial liver lesions are assigned stage III, and such lesions that are over 2 cm are assigned stage IIIC. Stage IIIA is consistent with microscopic abdominal metastasis, and stage IV includes liver parenchymal lesions.

The patient above is optimally debulked (<1 cm residual disease). The recommendation made by the gynecologic oncologist is that she undergo chemotherapy.

2. Such mode of chemotherapy is called

A. Primary chemotherapy

B. Adjuvant therapy

C. Neoadjuvant therapy

D. Salvage therapy

B Adjuvant chemotherapy is the use of drugs to treat patients who have undergone surgery as the initial therapeutic intervention. Neoadjuvant chemotherapy involves the use of chemotherapy prior to surgical reduction of tumor volume. Salvage chemotherapy is the use of a second-line therapy based on clinical or CA-125 criteria.

3. The recommended chemotherapeutic regimen for this patient is

A. Carboplatin and paclitaxel

B. Cisplatin and paclitaxel

C. EMA-CO

D. Carboplatin and cyclophosphamide

A Carboplatin and paclitaxel is the recommended adjuvant therapy for ovarian cancer patients. Although studies have shown cisplatin and paclitaxel to be equally effective, the side effects and the cost of administration of this regimen preclude it from being the first-line recommended therapy.

4. A 70-year-old woman with MMMT of the ovary is getting salvage therapy with ifosfamide. On day 3 of therapy, she complains of noting bright red spots upon wiping herself after urinating. All of the following are true about ifosfamide, *except:*

A. Ifosfamide is an alkylating agent that requires activation via the hepatic microsomal enzyme system.

B. Hemorrhagic cystitis is a common toxicity of this therapy and can be potentially prevented by using mesna.

C. CNS toxicity manifested as somnolence, lethargy, ataxia, confusion, disorientation, dizziness, malaise, and/or coma can be treated with methylene blue.

D. Smaller doses are required to achieve equivalent efficacy similar to cyclophosphamide.

D Just like cyclophosphamide, ifosfamide requires activation via the hepatic enzyme system. However, ifosfamide is activated more slowly than cyclophosphamide and forms proportionally less active alkylating agent. Therefore, larger doses are required for equivalent efficacy because more is excreted in the urine when compared with cyclophosphamide.

5. A 58-year-old woman is found to have recurrent endometrial carcinoma. Previously, she has been treated with surgery and whole pelvic radiation. Now, she is noted to have vaginal metastases and is recommended to undergo vaginal brachytherapy.

All of the following are true of brachytherapy, *except:*

A. External-beam radiation is used to focus the radiation toward the vagina.

B. The dose at a given distance from the source is determined largely by the inverse square law.

C. The amount of radiation administered via vaginal brachytherapy is calculated with respect to points A and B.

D. The radiation device is placed either within or close to the target tumor volume.

A Teletherapy is external-beam radiation. Linear accelerators are used while the patient is in either prone or supine position. Brachytherapy uses radiation applicators, such as intrauterine tandems or colpostats, to deliver radiation in close proximity to the tumor.

6. Following brachytherapy treatment, patient presents to the clinic with complaints of foul smelling discharge per vagina. You perform a quick tampon test in the clinic and it is positive. You have now diagnosed her with a vesicovaginal fistula. Rectovaginal or vesicovaginal fistulas are possible long-term complications of pelvic irradiation (3% to 6% incidence). Conservative management of fistulas may include all of the following, *except:*

A. Percutaneous nephrostomies

B. Bowel rest

C. Ureteral stents

D. Gracilis muscle flap

E. TPN therapy

D Vesicovaginal fistulas and ureteral strictures are possible long-term complications of radiation therapy. Bowel rest, placement of nephrostomies, insertion of ureteral stents, and TPN therapy are conservative measures that can be taken before surgical intervention, such as creating a gracilis muscle flap.

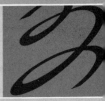

47

Palliative Care

Colleen McCormick

1. Which of the following interventions has not been shown to decrease pain from bone metastasis?

A. Radiation

B. Surgical fixation of pathologic fractures

C. Bisphosphonates

D. Calcitonin

> **D** Localized radiation treatment provides pain relief in 35% to 100% of patients with bone metastasis. Surgical fixation is appropriate for fractures. Bisphosphonates have been shown to decrease the rate of skeletal metastasis, and some studies support their use to decrease bone pain associated with metastasis. Calcitonin has not been shown to relieve bone pain from metastasis.

2. When converting to fentanyl patches from another form of narcotic, the previous narcotics should be

A. Stopped immediately

B. Continued for 2 hours after the patch is placed, then stopped

C. Continued for 12 hours after the patch is placed, then stopped

D. Continued for 24 hours after the patch has been applied, then stopped

C Narcotic converters are available to switch between narcotics. When changing between medications, the dose should be decreased by 25% to 50% to account for incomplete cross tolerance. Fentanyl can be converted 1:1 from IV to transdermal, and the IV can be tapered off with two steps over 12 hours. Note the importance that transdermal absorption requires more time than oral or intravenous routes, so medications must be continued after the fentanyl patch is started. However, these medications should not be continued at their previous level beyond the 12 hours required for transdermal absorption, or overdosing can result.

3. A patient with spinal metastasis and increasing leg weakness should be treated immediately with

   A. Solu-Medrol 10 mg IV
   B. Solu-Medrol 100 mg IV
   C. Dilantin

   B Epidural spinal cord compression from metastasis needs to be recognized, diagnosed, and treated rapidly to avoid permanent paralysis. Cord compression presents initially as pain, which is usually worse when lying down, and then progresses to weakness and hyperreflexia. Loss of bladder and bowel function and paralysis follows. An MRI should be obtained on all cancer patients with back pain, which can be treated with opiates and steroids. Steroids both relieve pain and decrease the rate of neurologic complications and can be given as a low or high regimen. The low dose regimen is 10 mg load then 16 mg a day, tapered over 2 weeks. If evidence of neurologic compromise exists, the high dose regimen should be used: 100 mg IV load then 24 mg tid for 3 days then tapered over 10 days. Antiseizure prophylaxis is not required for spinal metastasis.

48

HIV in Pregnancy

Catherine Eppes

1. When pregnant women are treated antenatally with highly active anti-retroviral therapy (HAART), which of the following most closely approximates the vertical transmission rate?

   A. 20% to 30%

   B. 10%

   C. 4%

   D. 1% to 2%

> **D** Patients treated with HAART therapy have a 1% to 2% vertical transmission rate. HAART therapy includes two nucleoside reverse transcriptase inhibitors plus either a protease inhibitor, a boosted protease inhibitor, or a nonnucleoside reverse transcriptase inhibitor, or three nonnucleoside reverse transcriptase inhibitors. All HAART medications should be started and stopped at the same time to reduce the emergence of viral resistance. Untreated patients have a 20% to 30% transmission rate, whereas those treated with zidovudine monotherapy have a 10% rate, and those treated with dual therapy have a 4% transmission rate.

2. Which group of pregnant women should be treated with anti-retroviral therapy?

   A. All pregnant women

   B. Those with CD4 counts less then 350

   C. Those with viral loads greater than 100,000

   D. Those who were previously on HAART

The guidelines for nonpregnant and pregnant adults differ. Although the initiation of antiretroviral therapy in nonpregnant individuals is typically delayed until plasma RNA levels of HIV exceed 100,000 or the CD4 count is less then 350, all pregnant women should be offered the opportunity to start antiretroviral therapy due to the reduction in vertical transmission.

3. A 35-year-old gravida 7 para 2042 at 37 4/7 weeks' gestation with HIV and a viral load of 1,100 presents 6 hours after having spontaneous rupture of her membranes. She is dilated 3 cm and 80% effaced. She was scheduled for a cesarean section at 38 weeks. Which of the following is the appropriate management?

A. Administer a loading dose of intravenous zidovudine and then proceed to cesarean section.

B. Administer the loading dose of zidovudine and then start Pitocin. She may deliver vaginally as long as rapid labor ensues.

C. Proceed to emergent cesarean section.

D. A and B

E. All of the above

D ACOG guidelines recommend scheduled cesarean sections in all women who have HIV RNA levels greater than 1,000 copies/mL before the onset of labor. Elective cesarean sections have been found to decrease the vertical transmission rates by 50%. However, studies have not shown benefit in women with HIV RNA copies less than 1,000 copies/mL. Therefore, these women can deliver vaginally. The benefit of a cesarean section after rupture of membranes or once labor has started is unknown. Therefore, the approach to delivery should be individualized. Intravenous zidovudine should be administered 3 hours before cesarean section. In this scenario, either option A or B is feasible. Because the patient has ruptured her membranes, whether a cesarean section would benefit is unknown. Notably, women with HIV appear to have more post cesarean complications, particularly if their CD4 count is less than 200.

4. A 23-year-old P0020 at 29 weeks is HIV-positive and has a CD4 count of 500. She is taking HAART, including a protease inhibitor. What is a common side effect?

A. Bacterial pneumonia

B. Hyperglycemia

C. Neural tube defects

D. Hepatotoxicity

> **B** Hyperglycemia is a recognized side effect of protease inhibitors, and a theoretic risk of increased incidence of diabetes and diabetic ketoacidosis is present. Other side effects that have been found include preterm labor (found in the Swiss Mother and Child HIV cohort but later meta-analysis did not find this association) and intrauterine growth restriction. Bacterial pneumonia and allergic reactions at the injection site are side effects reported in fusion inhibitors, a new class of medication used in those with multidrug resistance. Neural tube defects have been found in patients taking Sustiva (efavirenz) during the first trimester. Long-term usage of nevirapine has been associated with severe hepatotoxicity, including lethal hepatic necrosis in those with CD4 counts above 250.

5. All of the following should be avoided in pregnancy, *except:*

A. Efavirenz

B. Nevirapine

C. Retrovir

D. Delavirdine

> **C** All of the following, except Retrovir, should be avoided in pregnancy. Efavirenz has been linked to neural tube defects; nevirapine has been associated with hepatotoxicity, particularly in women with CD4 counts greater then $250/mm^3$. Delavirdine has not been studied well and therefore should be avoided. Retrovir (or zidovudine) has been associated with a 68% reduction in the rate of perinatal transmission.

6. Which of the following exhibits minimal transplacental passage?

A. Nucleoside reverse transcriptase inhibitors

B. Nonnucleoside reverse transcriptase inhibitors

C. Protease inhibitors

> **C** Nucleoside reverse transcriptase inhibitors are the most extensively studied class of drug in pregnancy, and both these and nonnucleoside reverse transcriptase inhibitors cross the placenta. Protease inhibitors exhibit minimal placental passage, and lower drug serum levels are reported during pregnancy.